CONTENTS

WITNESSES

TUESDAY, SEPTEMBER 24, 2002

ALPHABETICAL LIST OF WITNESSES

IV

APPENDIX

S. Hrg. 107–845

RESPONDING TO THE PUBLIC HEALTH THREAT OF WEST NILE VIRUS

JOINT HEARING

BEFORE THE

OVERSIGHT OF GOVERNMENT MANAGEMENT, RESTRUCTURING, AND THE DISTRICT OF COLUMBIA SUBCOMMITTEE

OF THE

COMMITTEE ON GOVERNMENTAL AFFAIRS UNITED STATES SENATE

AND THE

COMMITTEE ON HEALTH, EDUCATION, LABOR, AND PENSIONS

ONE HUNDRED SEVENTH CONGRESS

SECOND SESSION

SEPTEMBER 24, 2002

Printed for the use of the Committee on Governmental Affairs

U.S. GOVERNMENT PRINTING OFFICE

83–479 PDF   WASHINGTON : 2003

For sale by the Superintendent of Documents, U.S. Government Printing Office
Internet: bookstore.gpo.gov   Phone: toll free (866) 512–1800; DC area (202) 512–1800
Fax: (202) 512–2250   Mail: Stop SSOP, Washington, DC 20402–0001

COMMITTEE ON GOVERNMENTAL AFFAIRS

JOSEPH I. LIEBERMAN, Connecticut, *Chairman*

CARL LEVIN, Michigan
DANIEL K. AKAKA, Hawaii
RICHARD J. DURBIN, Illinois
ROBERT G. TORRICELLI, New Jersey
MAX CLELAND, Georgia
THOMAS R. CARPER, Delaware
JEAN CARNAHAN, Missouri
MARK DAYTON, Minnesota

FRED THOMPSON, Tennessee
TED STEVENS, Alaska
SUSAN M. COLLINS, Maine
GEORGE V. VOINOVICH, Ohio
THAD COCHRAN, Mississippi
ROBERT F. BENNETT, Utah
JIM BUNNING, Kentucky
PETER G. FITZGERALD, Illinois

JOYCE A. RECHTSCHAFFEN, *Staff Director and Counsel*
RICHARD A. HERTLING, *Minority Staff Director*
DARLA D. CASSELL, *Chief Clerk*

OVERSIGHT OF GOVERNMENT MANAGEMENT, RESTRUCTURING, AND THE DISTRICT OF COLUMBIA SUBCOMMITTEE

RICHARD J. DURBIN, Illinois, *Chairman*

DANIEL K. AKAKA, Hawaii
ROBERT G. TORRICELLI, New Jersey
THOMAS R. CARPER, Delaware
JEAN CARNAHAN, Missouri
MARK DAYTON, Minnesota

GEORGE V. VOINOVICH, Ohio
TED STEVENS, Alaska
SUSAN M. COLLINS, Maine
THAD COCHRAN, Mississippi
PETER G. FITZGERALD, Illinois

MARIANNE CLIFFORD UPTON, *Staff Director and Chief Counsel*
MELANIE LEITNER, *Congressional Fellow, Senator Durbin*
ANDREW RICHARDSON, *Minority Staff Director*
THERESA PRYCH, *Minority Legislative Aide*
BRIAN MCLAUGHLIN, *Staff Assistant*

COMMITTEE ON HEALTH, EDUCATION, LABOR, AND PENSIONS

EDWARD M. KENNEDY, Massachusetts, *Chairman*

CHRISTOPHER J. DODD, Connecticut
TOM HARKIN, Iowa
BARBARA A. MIKULSKI, Maryland
JAMES M. JEFFORDS (I), Vermont
JEFF BINGAMAN, New Mexico
PAUL D. WELLSTONE, Minnesota
PATTY MURRAY, Washington
JACK REED, Rhode Island
JOHN EDWARDS, North Carolina
HILLARY RODHAM CLINTON, New York

JUDD GREGG, New Hampshire
BILL FRIST, Tennessee
MICHAEL B. ENZI, Wyoming
TIM HUTCHINSON, Arkansas
JOHN W. WARNER, Virginia
CHRISTOPHER S. BOND, Missouri
PAT ROBERTS, Kansas
SUSAN M. COLLINS, Maine
JEFF SESSIONS, Alabama
MIKE DeWINE, Ohio

J. MICHAEL MYERS, *Staff Director and Chief Counsel*
TOWNSEND LANGE MCNITT, *Minority Staff Director*

RESPONDING TO THE PUBLIC HEALTH THREAT OF WEST NILE VIRUS

TUESDAY, SEPTEMBER 24, 2002

U.S. SENATE,
SUBCOMMITTEE ON OVERSIGHT OF GOVERNMENT MAN-
AGEMENT, RESTRUCTURING, AND THE DISTRICT OF CO-
LUMBIA, OF THE COMMITTEE ON GOVERNMENTAL AF-
FAIRS, AND THE COMMITTEE ON HEALTH, EDUCATION,
LABOR, AND PENSIONS,

Washington, DC.

The Committees met jointly, pursuant to notice, at 9:43 a.m., in room SD–342, Dirksen Senate Office Building, Hon. Richard Durbin, Chairman of the Subcommittee, presiding.

Present: Senators Durbin, Kennedy, Dodd, Landrieu, Carper, Reed, Gregg, Frist, Warner, Hutchinson, and Fitzgerald.

OPENING STATEMENT OF SENATOR DURBIN

Senator DURBIN. Good morning. The hearing will come to order. I want to thank my colleague, Senator Kennedy, for joining me. This is a joint hearing between our two Committees, from the Governmental Affairs Committee, which tries to help coordinate the agencies of government, and, of course, Senator Kennedy is Chairman of the Committee on Health, Education, Labor, and Pensions. It is a joint hearing on responding to the public health threat of the West Nile Virus.

What we have learned this summer is that mosquitoes can do more than ruin a backyard barbecue. For some Americans, particularly the elderly and medically vulnerable, that harmless mosquito bite can turn out to be life threatening. The numbers of American victims of West Nile Virus have not reached a level to rival major public health threats like influenza or measles, but the trend line is not encouraging.

Last year, there were 66 infections across America and 9 deaths from West Nile Virus as they were reported. This year, 1,963 infections have been reported. The death toll has reached 94. This morning, 2 more deaths were reported in my home State of Illinois, which has reached a total of 27, and for inexplicable reasons leads the Nation. In 1 year, the West Nile Virus infection rate is up almost 2,000 percent and fatalities over 1,000 percent.

The source of the virus could be in backyards and parks across America, despite the best efforts of the public health community. Particularly worrisome are the latest reports from Federal agencies that the virus can survive in the bloodstream and is likely then transmitted by organ donations and blood transfusions.

(1)

Today's hearing is the first in the Senate since the West Nile Virus truly became a national challenge. We will ask the experts in public health from Washington and across the Nation to give us an honest and accurate appraisal of this public health threat. We will ask the experts who monitor our Nation's blood supply what more we can do to guarantee its safety. We will learn the steps that are being taken to develop a vaccine to protect us. And most importantly, we will call on public health leaders from every level to develop a national strategy to reverse the trend of West Nile infection and mortality.

We had hoped for a break in the battle against West Nile Virus as the mosquito season winds down in most places across America, but the threats to our blood supply tell us this dangerous legacy may, and I underline "may," now threaten us year-round. The experts will tell us exactly what the threat may be.

We owe it to the families across our Nation to redouble our efforts to protect our Nation's blood supply and to prepare for the battle which awaits us again next year. Our two panels of witnesses will spell out the challenge and share with us their views on meeting it.

I would now like to turn to my colleague, Senator Kennedy, and ask him for his opening statement.

OPENING STATEMENT OF SENATOR KENNEDY

Senator KENNEDY. Thank you, Senator Durbin. I want to thank you very much for having this joint Committee hearing with us. Senator Durbin has been a real leader on this issue, which is of such enormous concern to families across this country and we welcome a chance to join with you today in helping us all, not only in the Congress, the American people, better understand the nature of the challenge that we are facing, as well as the kind of response that we are having and what more we can do to provide help and assistance to families across this country, and also to anticipate future kinds of challenges that are similar, as well, whether it's going to be in the food supply, where we're importing a great deal more, or other areas, as well.

So this hearing is very important, and I know Senator Durbin feels strongly and join with Senator Dodd that this is not just a hearing, it is the beginning of a very careful oversight, working with the administration where we can, trying to point up areas in which we need to make further progress.

Also, as I understand, we will be joined by Senator Breaux and Senator Landrieu of Louisiana, a State that has been particularly hard hit by the grim disease.

The goal of our hearing is to determine whether all necessary steps are being taken by Federal, State, and local governments to assist communities afflicted by the West Nile fever. Millions of Americans have now become aware that the West Nile fever can cause sickness and death. Recent reports show that the disease can cause symptoms similar to those of polio and can imperil the safety of the blood supply. That is an enormously important issue. We want to hear from our leaders to better understand and to guide us on the policies. We have important questions about the blood supply and its safety. We want to hear from our witnesses on this issue.

In a few short weeks, the virus has spread from the Atlantic to the Pacific, from border to border. Congress should do all it can to protect the American people from this emerging health threat. We should provide the adequate funding for public health measures to contain and reduce the spread of the disease. We should expedite the development of vaccine through new investments in research.

Threats to our Nation come in many forms. In the war against disease, the battlegrounds will be our Nation's emergency rooms and the heroes will be our Nation's health care professionals. To win this war, we need to restore the funding for hospitals, invest in the training of doctors and nurses, and to rebuild our public health capacity. The price of victory may be high, but the cost of defeat is higher still.

The newspapers even yesterday were pointing out the very great amount of pressure that is on the government, the pressures that are on our hospitals, and about the crowding. On the front page of the *Washington Post* yesterday, we are talking about the crowding in the hospitals, crowding in the emergency room, crowding in the operating rooms. We have the stories in our national newspapers now where we are having further proposal by the administration of cuts in the support of our health care systems. The hospitals are the first line of defense, the public health system in order to detect it, and then the hospitals to contain it, and we know about the serious cutbacks that the administration is involved in now.

So we have all got an important responsibility if we are talking about trying to deal with this, to make sure that we are going to give the support to the hospitals and to the professional personnel that are so necessary to deal with this issue.

In the bioterrorism legislation enacted into law earlier this year, we have begun to make some of the investments necessary to protect against deadly diseases. These investments are needed more than ever to prevent the spread of West Nile fever. In fact, our public health infrastructure had deteriorated so significantly that the initial diagnosis of disease was needlessly delayed. We are going to need a strong public health system if we are going to meet our responsibilities to the Nation's people on the whole issue on bioterrorism, as well as the kind of challenge that we are facing with West Nile.

Unfortunately, the administration's budget steps back when it comes to protecting the public health. While purporting to provide more funding to hospitals to strengthen public health and combat bioterrorism, the President's budget actually cuts funding to America's hospitals. We cannot afford to keep Americans well and protect the public health if the administration will not do its part.

We have already seen what can be accomplished through resolute action to meet a public health challenge. Within the last year, funds and leadership provided by Congress, working in partnership with the administration, produced an effective national response to smallpox, and I am proud that a Massachusetts company is leading the way in producing a new and safer vaccine for the dread disease. We should show the same resolve in responding to the threat of West Nile.

A few years ago, few Americans other than the specialists in exotic diseases had even heard of West Nile Virus. Today, it is a disease familiar to households across the Nation. The virus was first detected in New York in 1999. In the next 2 years, the disease caused 18 deaths, 131 illnesses. This year alone, over 1,900 people across the United States have become ill and 94 have died. In just the last month, the number of cases has nearly doubled. Senior citizens in South Boston and senior citizens in Weymouth have died. This month, Massachusetts identified its first child case of West Nile, something the State had never, never seen before.

We need to determine whether the steps now being taken by the Centers for Disease Control are adequate to halt the spread of this disease and minimize the severity of the illness it causes. Basic public health precautions, such as using insect repellents, and eliminating standing water near homes can reduce infections. CDC is working with local communities to provide public health information about proper precautions, but infection rates continue to rise. Clearly, we must do more.

We also need to determine whether the FDA and the other public health agencies are taking proper steps to protect the safety of the blood supply and transplanted organs and whether NIH is developing the new vaccines, therapies, and diagnostic tests as rapidly as possible to prevent infection and to protect the health of those affected by West Nile.

As significant as the threat of West Nile fever itself is today, it may also be a sign of even more deadly outbreaks in the years to come. In this era of global jet travel, it is possible to have breakfast in a country half a world away and arrive in the United States for dinner. We also import millions of tons of food from around the world. Whether released deliberately by a terrorist, like the lethal anthrax attacks of last year—I draw a distinction. Whether we are facing the possibility of a terrorist, or the kind of a lethal anthrax attacks of last year, or brought to our country accidentally, deadly infections will threaten our health security for many years to come.

Our hearing today will consider how we are responding to the West Nile fever today and also how we respond to other deadly disease outbreaks in the years to come. I thank Senator Durbin for Co-Chairing this joint hearing and look forward to the witnesses.

I especially want to welcome Julie Gerberding. This will be her first appearance in the Senate with assuming her new responsibilities in a long and distinguished career. So we very much welcome her as well as the other witnesses, and I thank the Chair.

Senator DURBIN. Thank you, Senator Kennedy. Senator Gregg.

OPENING STATEMENT OF SENATOR GREGG

Senator GREGG. Thank you, Senator Durbin and Senator Kennedy, for holding this hearing on the West Nile Virus issue, which is an issue that is of immediate and significant importance to many of us, especially on the East Coast and as it moves toward the West Coast.

We have had, as Senator Kennedy has mentioned, a large expansion of this virus. We are now seeing it in my State. Senator Kennedy mentioned the unfortunate deaths in Massachusetts. We are seeing in my State the death of the bird population, which is clearly tied to the West Nile Virus infection, and the fact that that could be transmitted to humans in Northern New England. It has already caused, I believe, close to 94 deaths in our country and there have been 1,700 human cases of West Nile, in the country, and so we need to address the issue.

Some of the concerns have been outlined by Senator Kennedy. I think my concerns go to a couple of other areas. First, I am interested in knowing the origins of the disease. I would like to know that for the very obvious reason that if we know the origin of the disease, maybe we can stop other diseases of the same type and potency from coming into the country if we have a sense of what the origin of the disease is.

Second, I am interested in knowing what the effect of spraying is on the mosquito population, specifically whether the benefits of spraying are outweighed by the negative impacts of spraying. Obviously, we have known for years that certain types of spraying do have a significant environmental impact. Is it appropriate for us, however, to initiate an aggressive spraying program in the face of those environmental impacts because the human impact of not doing the spraying is more significant? Even though our witnesses are not from the environmental community, I would be interested in hearing their comments on that.

And third, and probably of most significance is the issue of our blood supply and how we maintain the integrity of our blood supply in light of the virus, which appears to be a potential threat to that blood supply.

These are big issues. They are big issues for us from a public policy standpoint and obviously from a public health standpoint and I certainly appreciate the Chairman holding these hearings and bringing forward these excellent witnesses so that we can get some information out to the public on this question. Thank you.

Senator DURBIN. Thanks, Senator Gregg. Senator Dodd.

OPENING STATEMENT OF SENATOR DODD

Senator DODD. Very briefly, Mr. Chairman. I think you have covered the ground and Senator Kennedy and Senator Gregg have raised some very appropriate questions. I am obviously anxious to hear from our witnesses.

As Senator Gregg and Senator Kennedy has pointed out, I guess those of us from the East Coast feel this more pointedly because it has been around now since 1999 for all of us, though obviously it is moving across the country and indications on the very West Coast are that there are some cases that have sprung up. So we are very interested in getting an answer to this.

There is nothing more intimidating or frightening to people than to have something apparently almost as innocent as a mosquito, although history has shown how lack of innocence a mosquito can have, but certainly in recent times, relative innocence and bringing such hardship. So I am very interested in hearing what our witnesses have to say.

I think it is important at the hearing here we also commend, however, the Centers for Disease Control, NIH, the FDA, as well, who have been working pretty hard on this, our State and locals. We received $200,000 in Connecticut already in this area. We have not had a human life lost. We have had a number of cases identified in our State, so it is a growing concern.

This is a very important hearing and I commend both of the Chairs for bringing two committees together. This is a wonderful example of how committees can work together with somewhat overlapping jurisdiction to try and address an issue like this.

I also want to underscore the point Senator Kennedy made here. It is one that needs to be made, and that is while the answer here is not just writing the check, it obviously does take investment of resources. That $200,000 that my State received from the Federal Government has been awfully important to my State, particularly in times when we are facing huge budget deficits. And so when people out there talk about homeland security, obviously we narrow that definition to some degree, but certainly if you ask the average citizen in our country whether or not they think this is an issue that deserves an aggressive action on the part of local, State, and Federal Government, I think the answer would be a resounding yes, before this gets totally out of control and we find ourselves in a far more difficult situation.

I want to underscore that point, that as we look at these issues and our budgets, obviously, this is an important one. It certainly is in our State. Pick up the morning paper here in Washington, DC this morning and ask the people of Virginia whether or not they think this is an important matter, having lost another life.

So I thank you and I look forward to the testimony.

Senator DURBIN. Thanks, Senator Dodd.

I learned this morning of two more deaths in Illinois, one in Peoria and one in Chicago. Again, as I mentioned at the outset, for some reason, our State is leading the Nation in this. As you mention, it started on the East Coast. The infection has now been found in 41 States and the District of Columbia, so it is truly a national challenge.

Let me welcome the first panel. Dr. Julie Gerberding, thank you, the new Director of the Centers for Disease Control and Prevention, the Federal agency charged with coordinating our national response to the West Nile Virus. Dr. Anthony Fauci, truly a leader in public health and world recognized and respected, Director of the National Institute of Allergy and Infectious Diseases at the National Institutes of Health. He is going to discuss the ongoing biomedical research related to the West Nile Virus. And Dr. Jesse Goodman, who is the Deputy Director of the Food and Drug Administration, Center for Biologics Evaluation and Research, who is focusing on the threat of the West Nile Virus to the safety of our blood supply.

Thank you for joining us. It is customary in our Subcommittee to swear in all witnesses and I would ask you to please stand.

Do you solemnly swear the testimony you are about to give is the truth, the whole truth, and nothing but the truth, so help you, God?

Dr. GERBERDING. I do.

Dr. FAUCI. I do.

Dr. GOODMAN. I do.

Senator DURBIN. Thank you. The record will indicate that the witnesses have answered in the affirmative.

I would ask you each to give us, if you can, in 5 minutes, a summary of this challenge as you see it. We may have colleagues coming in from time to time. We are facing a 10:30 vote, so we are trying to get the first panel's testimony in before that and we would appreciate any help you could give us in reaching that goal.

Dr. Gerberding, please commence.

TESTIMONY OF JULIE LOUISE GERBERDING, M.D., M.P.H.,[1] DIRECTOR, CENTERS FOR DISEASE CONTROL AND PREVENTION, U.S. DEPARTMENT OF HEALTH AND HUMAN SERVICES

Dr. GERBERDING. Good morning and thank you. Thank you, Mr. Chairman, thank you, Chairman Kennedy, Senator Dodd, Senator Gregg, and all of the Members of the Committee. It is a great privilege for me to be here in my first appearance before Congress as the Director of the CDC and the Administrator of ATSDR and I really first want to thank you for all the support that you have given CDC and ATSDR in our work in public health over the last many years, both here in the United States but also internationally.

We are 600 miles away from Washington, but not out of sight, and we would certainly welcome you visiting CDC in Atlanta and would, of course, like to visit you in your own States, as well, but really would like to show you the progress that we have made, the first steps, at least, in rebuilding the public health infrastructure, in large part because of the support this Committee has given us. I think we can convince you that we are accountable for those investments and really have made some important progress.

Today's topic is, of course, West Nile, which really is a prime example of an emerging infectious disease. So all of the infrastructure and all of the components of public health really have to come to bear to help us identify and respond to this new emerging infectious problem in the United States. It is also an excellent example of how the investments that we have made in the bioterrorism infrastructure have assisted us in responding to other public health threats, as well, and I will get back to that in a moment.

As of this morning, there were 1,965 human cases of West Nile Virus reported from 32 States and Washington, DC. At least 94 of these patients have died. Our concern for the human toll of this disease is enormous. Clearly, it is not a problem just for the people who have been diagnosed with the more severe forms of the illness, but for every case of severe encephalitis, there are 150 additional people who have been infected, and about 20 percent of those have milder symptoms of the disease. So it is having an enormous impact on all of us.

I will just say, I have had personal experience with this in my own backyard. My husband acquired West Nile infection, fortunately a mild case, but we experienced firsthand how alarming and how disturbing this illness can really be.

This is a mosquito-borne disease. It was first diagnosed in Uganda in 1937, and since that time, it has been the cause of numerous outbreaks in the Middle East and Eastern Europe. Over the last 10 years, those outbreaks have been conspicuous in Russia, Roma-

---

[1] The prepared statement of Dr. Gerberding appears in the Appendix on page 53.

nia, and Israel, and the new finding in the last decade has been the association of those infections with the severe neurologic disease.

The infection arrived in the United States in New York City in 1999, and you can see here in the blue the areas of the country that were involved with West Nile during 1999. In green, the spread in the year 2000 up and down the East Coast. In the pink, 2001, spread north, and then further into the central parts of the United States. And finally, this year, in yellow, the further extension to the West and to the South. I should also mention that we have cases in Canada. We are conducting surveillance in Mexico and are suspicious that we have got cases in Mexico, and as the mosquito vectors and the infected birds migrate North and South, we can only expect this pattern of progression to continue and we would anticipate a further extension next year into the West Coast.

The life cycle of this virus really moves between birds and mosquitoes. So the mosquitoes move the infection from one bird to another, and over the course of the summer, there is an acceleration of the concentration of the virus in the infected birds, so the mosquitoes become much more efficient at transmitting it.

On this graphic, you can see on the top the counties in the United States that have had human cases, including one human case in Los Angeles County. But in the middle, the counties that are reporting infections in birds. And finally, on the bottom, the counties that are reporting infections in horses. You see it is a tremendous burden of infection across the United States, concentrating this year predominately in the South, Louisiana, Mississippi, Alabama, and Arkansas, and then in the Midwest, particularly in Illinois, Michigan, Ohio, and the other Central States.

Where is this virus going to go? It is too soon to tell, but we know that it is following the pattern of birds and we can predict where the next human cases are going to be by doing the surveillance in the bird and animal population, because they do accurately predict where the next wave will be, and certainly, the information we need to target our integrated vector control programs.

So, in other words, when we see that the virus is active or there are dead birds in a particular area, then we can go in there and CDC will provide the technical support to that jurisdiction to initiate the appropriate steps to control the vector and also accelerate the information campaigns with the clinicians and the public health system and the people to ensure that the individual protective measures are being taken.

Those protection measures include eliminating, to the extent possible, standing water where mosquitoes breed. That is a very important component of this. But in addition, the advice to individuals to wear insect repellant that contains DEET when they do go outside, particularly in the evenings and the mornings when the most common mosquitoes involved in this feed. Also, to use proper screens on the windows and do the other kinds of things to help avoid mosquito bites.

One of the concerning aspects of this problem is that it is present in virtually all kinds of mosquitoes and all birds, so it is unlike some of the other vector-borne virus infections.

There are many prevention steps that we are taking, many more steps that need to continue, but I think we have made substantial progress. We are managing this outbreak through our Emergency Operations Center, the same way we managed anthrax through our Emergency Operations Center, and I think that helps us provide our coordination and communication functions, as well as the training and education of clinicians that are so vital to the detection and management of the patients.

We look forward to doing more, but I think this is a true example of the importance of a public health infrastructure and the integration with State and local partners, as well as our partners in the Federal Government through HHS and Secretary Thompson's leadership to really get this job done right, and we look forward to continuing to make progress. Thank you.

Senator GREGG. Mr. Chairman, could I just ask one clarifying point?

Senator DURBIN. Sure. Of course. Senator Gregg.

Senator GREGG. You said use mosquito repellant that included DEET.

Dr. GERBERDING. Correct. DEET is a mosquito repellant that keeps mosquitoes from attacking because they cannot find your scent. It comes in different concentrations. It needs to be present on the skin or on the clothing in order to serve as an effective repellant and it is the only mosquito repellant that we have documented evidence of efficacy for.

Senator GREGG. There was a fair amount of discussion in the last 10 years that people should not use DEET-based mosquito repellant.

Dr. GERBERDING. Well, I think the data that we have indicate that it is effective at preventing mosquito bites and we are not aware of any toxic effects in humans. For children, we recommend that very small infants not use it because their skin is more absorbent, and for pre-adolescent children that it not be used in a concentration higher than 10 percent. But we have not documented adverse health effects from using this product to date.

Senator GREGG. Thank you.

Senator DURBIN. Thanks, Senator Gregg. Dr. Fauci.

TESTIMONY OF ANTHONY FAUCI, M.D.,[1] DIRECTOR, NATIONAL INSTITUTE OF ALLERGY AND INFECTIOUS DISEASES, NATIONAL INSTITUTES OF HEALTH, U.S. DEPARTMENT OF HEALTH AND HUMAN SERVICES

Dr. FAUCI. Thank you very much, Mr. Chairman, Members of the Committee. It is a pleasure to be here with you this morning to talk about some of the research endeavors at NIH with regard to West Nile Virus.

I want to point out first that West Nile Virus is a member of the flavivirus family and we have been studying for years other related viruses as you see there, such as yellow fever, Japanese encephalitis, and dengue. So our ability to hit the ground running with regard to West Nile was really based on the fact that we have a program with flaviviruses that had gone on for years.

---

[1] The prepared statement of Dr. Fauci appears in the Appendix on page 57.

As you heard from Dr. Gerberding, there is a wide range of clinical manifestations with West Nile Virus. Although only one out of five individuals develop mild febrile disease and only one in 150 to 200 develop serious complications, there are many enigmas associated with what has been called the path of physiology of this disease, questions that we at NIH are directing our endeavors to.

Of note also, most fatal cases are in individuals greater than 50 years old. There is a very sharp dichotomy in case fatality rate and age, which is something we need to probe more closely because there are some important clues about the body's ability to handle infections in general, but particularly this infection related to age.

Now, with regard to the research agenda at NIH, it is divided into several directions, some of which we have already been quite successful in. First of all, as I mentioned, we are studying the basic research on the virus, which gives us many clues, not only in the disease itself, but also in the development of vaccines, diagnostics, and therapeutics. We are studying vector biology to ask some of the questions that Dr. Gerberding alluded to. Why, with this virus, is virtually every mosquito able to be a vector and what is the relationship between the vector, the intermediate hosts, and the primary hosts? We also have, obviously, a very intense effort in vaccine development, antiviral screening, which I will get into in a moment, and rapid diagnostics.

Some of the accomplishments that we have been able to achieve over the last year and a half to two, is the development of what we call a chimeric West Nile Virus vaccine, which is going to cut off the time requirement to get to a vaccine probably by several years. We screened over 300 drugs and we have about 15 hits of drugs that might be promising as direct antivirals.

We have a successful animal model, the golden hamster, which has allowed us to test the vaccine with direct challenges in an animal. Development of an animal model is critical in pursuing the pathogenesis and treatment of diseases.

We are, together with private companies as well as our sister agencies in the Public Health Service and the Department of Health and Human Services, working on rapid diagnostics.

And finally, we are responsible for the world reference center for arboviruses, which is a worldwide resource, so that when you have a new virus and vectors, you have a whole reference center that people can pull out and compare previous experiences.

This is the model that I was referring to. It is really quite interesting. We already have an attenuated yellow fever virus, which as I mentioned on the first poster is one of the flavivirus family. So what we are able to do is to take the genes of the coat protein of West Nile Virus and insert it into the genes of the already existing yellow fever vaccine to develop what we call a chimera that is what we say is a yellow fever backbone but is actually expressing the proteins of West Nile. That really does cut off several years in the process of vaccine development.

The company, Senator Kennedy, that is working on this is Acambis in Massachusetts and we are intramurally doing it also with dengue, so it is really quite promising.

The plans and the opportunities that we have, as many as we would have advances, there are as many unanswered questions, so our programs for the coming year will be directed at those. We are going to try and develop new products through expanded discovery.

Importantly is the immunity to West Nile Virus, including cross-reactivity. We found a very interesting finding in the animal model. If you infect the hamster with either yellow fever, St. Louis encephalitis, or dengue and they recover from it and then you challenge them with West Nile Virus, they are protected against West Nile Virus, which means the underlying immunity that you might even get from a yellow fever vaccination perhaps might give some degree of protection, which again is fortifying evidence why we are on the right track with the vaccine development.

Also, the human disease cases, the consequences and age dependence, why are we now seeing anterior horn disease similar to poliomyelitis? Why is there such a sharp age dependent discrepancy in mortality? These are all the future unanswered questions.

In addition, we are looking at immune-based therapies, interferon alpha, hyperimmune globulin, as well as some non-immune-based approaches. And finally, understanding the ecology of the host and the vectors.

So in summary, Members of the Committee, we belong, as Dr. Gerberding alluded to at the conclusion of her discussion, is that this is really part of the continuing spectrum of the threat of emerging and reemerging diseases, be they naturally occurring diseases or diseases that are deliberately perpetrated on society in the form of bioterrorism. It is all part of the program of understanding the relationship between emerging diseases and their human hosts. This falls right in the middle of it and is a cogent example of just yet another thing that we, the human species, have to face, from the flu pandemic of 1918 to the AIDS epidemic, which we are still in the middle of suffering from that, to know a new and reemerging disease. We will, according to what was said just a few moments ago, pool the resources of the Department of Health and Human Services and all the sister agencies to try and meet this challenge and hopefully protect the American public against future challenges. Thank you very much.

Thank you, Doctor.

Senator DURBIN. Dr. Goodman.

TESTIMONY OF JESSE L. GOODMAN, M.D., M.P.H.,[1] DEPUTY DIRECTOR, CENTER FOR BIOLOGICS EVALUATION AND RESEARCH, FOOD AND DRUG ADMINISTRATION, U.S. DEPARTMENT OF HEALTH AND HUMAN SERVICES

Dr. GOODMAN. Good morning, Mr. Chairman and Members of the Committees here. I am Jesse Goodman, an infectious disease physician and scientist and Deputy Director of the Center for Biologics Evaluation and Research at FDA. I thank you for providing FDA with the opportunity to speak with you here today about West Nile Virus.

As Dr. Fauci and Dr. Gerberding have said, there are, and, in fact, always will be, newly emerging infectious diseases which pose a threat to human health, and some of these will likely threaten

---

[1] The prepared statement of Dr. Goodman appears in the Appendix on page 60.

the safety of the blood supply. West Nile Virus is the newest of these such challenges.

In this testimony, I would like to do three things. First, I will provide a brief chronology of recent events from the perspective of blood safety. Second, I will tell you about what the response has been so far. And finally, I will tell you about our plans to further address the problem.

I think you will see that we have come a very long way in just three short weeks, and I would like to mention the extraordinary cooperation between CDC and FDA and the impressive pace with which the case investigations have been conducted. I would also like to thank the involved States and the blood organizations whose response to date has really been exemplary.

Until less than a month ago, the potential threat of West Nile Virus to the blood supply was thought to be very low. Because of the dramatic increase in the spread of West Nile Virus this year, on August 17, FDA, in consultation with CDC and NIH, issued an alert. This alert to the blood banks emphasized the importance of careful attention to screening procedures for blood donors, especially the exclusion of donors with even mild flu-like symptoms which could be early signs of West Nile Virus infection.

Then, about 3 weeks ago, the initial results of the investigation of a cluster of cases among the organ transplant recipients from a single organ donor led to strong suspicion that the virus could be transmitted by organ transplantation. We now believe it almost certain that the organs from a single donor carried the infections to four recipients. The source of the donor's infections may have been either natural, from mosquitoes, or from transfusions.

During our current state of heightened alert, several cases in which West Nile Virus disease developed in the days to weeks following a blood transfusion, both in and out of the setting of organ transplantation, have now been reported and are under investigation. In each case so far, the patients were from areas of known natural disease transmission.

However, as you have heard, special studies of blood donated to a single patient in Mississippi who later developed West Nile Virus disease suggested that three blood donors may have unwittingly and coincidentally had West Nile Virus in their blood at the time they donated. So far, one of these donors' infections has been confirmed.

Based on these ongoing investigations, we have identified a risk to blood safety, but I must caution you that we do not know at this time how big or small that risk may be. Critical studies are now being implemented in partnership with the other agencies, the States, the blood organizations, and in different donor populations to assess the risk to the blood and organ recipients in this country.

Meanwhile, we have taken several important steps. First, we are continuing to encourage the reporting of cases of West Nile Virus that follow recent transfusion or organ transplantation. If a case is reported in a recent donor, any blood products still available are being withdrawn.

Second, FDA is working with blood banks to improve the reporting of post-donation illnesses and appropriate actions to be taken, including withdrawal of products where needed to help protect others.

Third, because of the potential for West Nile Virus transmission by donors who never even develop any symptoms of infection, FDA believes it is important to be ready and able, if and when needed, to move rapidly towards screening testing of donor blood. No validated test is currently available for donor screening, and such screening of a large number of samples cannot be implemented overnight. However, I want to say there are some promising assays.

To jump start the process of getting to a reliable and practical diagnostic test, last week, we took the unusual and proactive step of meeting with the American Association of Blood Banks, AdvaMed (a Medical Diagnostics Device Manufacturing Association) and other partners in the blood banking and diagnostic testing industries, along with laboratories whose current tests could be potentially adapted to meet this need. CBER will also continue and, if necessary, expand its related work relevant to the development and review of potential West Nile Virus diagnostics, vaccines, and treatments, such as mentioned by Dr. Fauci.

I am pleased to report that the medical diagnostics and blood banking communities are highly engaged and motivated by the potential public health threat that we are now facing. While the success of these efforts depends largely on their overcoming scientific and technical obstacles, some of which may be significant, our hope is that, if needed, a West Nile Virus screening test for blood could become available, at least for study under investigation and new drug application, for the next transmission season.

At the same time, we are continuing to explore a relatively new strategy for treating blood to kill microbes called pathogen inactivation, and we are working with the developers of these technologies to help carefully assess their safety and determine whether they can be important in helping deal with West Nile Virus.

In conclusion, while we believe there is sufficient evidence to say there is a risk to the blood supply from West Nile Virus. We should keep this risk in perspective. There are approximately 4.5 million people in the United States who receive blood products each year. Both blood transfusion and organ transplantation are often life saving or life enhancing. While it is currently believed that the risk is low, it is important to say that our knowledge is very recent and is limited and it is changing rapidly. We believe patients should be aware that this risk exists and can discuss any concerns about their medical treatment and possible options with their physicians.

FDA, CDC, HRSA, and all of our partners are monitoring the situation. We will continue to work together to better understand and deal with the risk as quickly as possible.

Meanwhile, let me also take the opportunity to remind everyone that blood donation is a key to maintaining an adequate blood supply in our country, and regardless of the findings and concerns here, blood donation remains safe. Blood has been in short supply and we encourage and thank all the Americans who donate blood.

We have come a long way in a few short weeks, and I am optimistic that we can and will respond to this new challenge rapidly and effectively. Success in controlling the mosquito-borne epidemic itself will be critical in determining the risk of infection in the blood supply and the need for future blood screening.

Again, I thank you for the opportunity to be here today and welcome your questions.

Senator DURBIN. Thank you, Dr. Goodman.

We have many questions, and as I mentioned earlier, there is a vote on at 10:30. I see that two or three of my colleagues have joined us and I would like to ask them if they would not mind giving a very brief opening statement, perhaps 2 minutes or 3 minutes, and then we can go to the first questions. Let me start with Senator Frist, then Senator Landrieu, and Senator Warner.

OPENING STATEMENT OF SENATOR FRIST

Senator FRIST. Thank you, Mr. Chairman, and I thank all three of you for being here today and for your excellent presentations. All three of you have emphasized the importance of "dual use" of the resources that we, through government, make available to you—resources targeting bioterrorism as well as other public health threats.

By providing additional resources since September 11 to combat bioterrorism, your discussion of the response to West Nile Virus has been a good demonstration of such "dual use." With your chart, Dr. Fauci, you mention other public health threats—HIV/AIDS, West Nile Virus, and the flu. You could very easily add smallpox, which is on the front page of the paper, as well, in terms of the need to prevention, response, and surveillance, as we go forward. So over the course of the morning, I would be interested in both this panel and the next panel commenting further on how we can address strengthening our public health infrastructure to address all of these public health threats.

The spread of West Nile Virus started in 1999. We see where we are today. Dr. Goodman, you said we have no screening test for West Nile Virus, and we essentially have no treatment today. Additionally, the virus is in our blood supply, to some extent. The viral contamination of the blood supply can strike great fear in people's hearts and minds, and it shows there is a lot to be done.

Knowing the natural history of such a disease, did we respond as quickly as we should have over the last 3 years. What do we expect in the next month? Due to the cooling weather, the risk of transmission through the mosquitoes is linked. Is West Nile Virus going to disappear, or is it going to come back with a bigger surge next year?

Senator DURBIN. Thank you, Senator Frist. Senator Landrieu, if you would like to make an opening statement.

OPENING STATEMENT OF SENATOR LANDRIEU

Senator LANDRIEU. Very briefly, Mr. Chairman. Thank you for calling this hearing. It is very timely, and as you know, the most cases of West Nile Virus have been in the Chairman's State, Illinois, but Louisiana is second, with 11 deaths and over 260 people infected. In our capital city in Louisiana, we reported 3 deaths and 42 people ill. So while this is a very serious situation everywhere, it is particularly urgent in Louisiana.

Mr. Chairman and Members, I am very pleased that one of our parish presidents is here with us, Nickie Monica of St. John Parish, who will be testifying as part of the second panel.

Louisiana has been spraying for mosquitoes since the very first person landed in Louisiana over 300 years ago, trying to get rid of these pests, and up until recently, that is what they were, pests. It is extremely aggravating and in some ways debilitating to be working in a place where mosquitoes can be serious pests, but never before have we faced this kind of illness that can bring with it death. People are very concerned.

My point would only be today that while we focus Federal help on the disease itself, on the infection and the treatment, let us remember who is on the front lines, our parish and county officials, trying to get funding for the spraying to prevent the spread by mosquitoes. We cannot, I think, lose sight of the need that our local officials have just for the eradication of the carriers of this deadly disease, the mosquito.

So I thank the panel. I am looking forward to hearing from you all. Thank you, Mr. Chairman, for calling this hearing today.

Senator DURBIN. Senator Landrieu, thank you.

Senator Warner, I know you saw this morning's paper.

OPENING STATEMENT OF SENATOR WARNER

Senator WARNER. Yes. This is our paper today. I point out it is front page news showing the depth of the concern, as pointed out by our colleague, Senator Landrieu. When the question comes, I hope you would share with us what knowledge you may have, apart from the scientific. We gained the clear impression everything can be done by the organizations, State and Federal, who have jurisdiction over problems like this, but what about advice to the citizens on how they might alter their daily activities, themselves and their children, to minimize this? The obvious, of course, is at twilight, when the mosquitoes are most active, get indoors, I suppose. Simple things like that would be helpful.

Senator DURBIN. Thank you, Senator. Is there anything further you would like to add?

Senator WARNER. No.

Senator DURBIN. What we are going to try to do is this. I am going to ask Senator Kennedy and Senator Gregg to ask the first round of questions, and if a vote starts, I will take off and try to make that vote and return so that we can just keep this moving apace. But let me open with Senator Kennedy's opportunity.

Senator KENNEDY. Thank you very much. Thank you.

Let me ask you, do you think there is any way to eradicate the West Nile or are we stuck with this every summer from now on?

Dr. GERBERDING. The pattern of the similar viruses in this family is that they wax and wane over years, but we can never really completely eradicate them from the population because they are just too deeply embedded between the birds and the mosquitoes. As we over-winter, meaning the mosquitoes in the Southern part of the United States do not die off in the winter, so they may continue to transmit all year round, it is just about impossible to completely eliminate it.

Senator KENNEDY. Is there anything that you can tell us about whether it is rising or declining? What can we anticipate for the next year, next summer, the summer after? What does your analysis reflect on this?

Dr. GERBERDING. In terms of this year, in the Southern States, the epidemic started very early and has already peaked and is beginning to fade away. In the Northern States, especially around the Great Lakes, it started much later, much more rapid increase in cases, but there, too, we are beginning to see a decline suggesting that this year's epidemic is beginning to wane off. And, of course, as the weather gets cold up North, we would expect to see a marked reduction in cases because the mosquitoes would no longer be feeding.

Senator KENNEDY. One of the few advantages of the colder winter.

Dr. GERBERDING. That is right.

Senator KENNEDY. But in any event, what it is for next year, it is difficult to anticipate whether it is going to be more virulent next year during the spring and the summer? It is difficult to tell?

Dr. GERBERDING. It is very difficult to tell because, in part, it depends on the weather, and it also depends on the micro-climate. The West Coast is very different from the South, but it also depends on to what extent we get out there early on with the integrated control programs and deal with larvacides and also the extent to which people implement their own personal protective measures.

Senator KENNEDY. Dr. Fauci, you mentioned the development of a vaccine. How close are we to the development of a vaccine on this?

Dr. FAUCI. The phase one trial, where we put it into humans and start determining safety, are going to be underway imminently. Hopefully, what we will have is about a year's worth of that and then go right into phase two. So I would imagine it is 3 or so years away, which is really light speed when you are thinking in terms of the development of a vaccine. So we will likely have one, if successful, within the next few years.

Senator KENNEDY. What will that mean for people, that they will be able to take it and be immunized to the disease, is that right?

Dr. FAUCI. The same say, since it is a flavivirus, as I pointed out, the same way when you get a yellow fever vaccination. You are essentially protected from yellow fever if you go on a trip to a yellow fever endemic area. It might turn out, depending on the evolution of the epidemic, that we would take at-risk people, particularly people who are immunosuppressed or people who are beyond a certain age, and they will be the first targets of a vaccine program.

Senator KENNEDY. Dr. Goodman, you mentioned that you have been meeting with the blood banks and those that have been involved in that industry, that they are motivated. If needed, you could mandate a test, but you are looking at other tests that may be helpful in terms of dealing with the pathogens, I guess, in the total blood supply.

But why should we not mandate a test now? The idea, as I understand it, is that you mandate the test, it builds up the interest from those that may be interested in producing a test and it only goes in effect when they develop it, but it creates the market. It creates the financial incentives for those to go in there.

Given the evidence that we have in terms of the blood supply, I heard you when you said that it may not stay in the blood supply for a very long time, but we have seen this infection expand. For the people that are going to be endangered, that is not a very good, satisfactory answer. Why not go ahead and mandate the test now?

Dr. GOODMAN. Well, I think it is a good question and what we have signaled very strongly to the diagnostics industry and the blood community is that based on this rapidly evolving evidence we are seeing, that we think it is very likely that there will be a need to do generalized testing of blood.

Senator KENNEDY. Let me stop you there. What does it mean to people that are watching this, it looks like the development, that there may be a reason that we go in to try and may do this in the future, I mean, these are as current as this hearing. People are out there and they are concerned. When we can go ahead and mandate this test, why do we not just go ahead and make this a matter of public policy? Why not just go ahead and do that?

Dr. GOODMAN. First of all, we are proceeding as if generalized testing of the blood will be needed, so in that sense, I totally agree with you. In terms of mandating——

Senator KENNEDY. Excuse me, and I want to give you a chance to finish. The generalized test that you are looking at is in a much broader kind of scope, to look at a variety of different things rather than just the West Nile.

Dr. GOODMAN. Oh, no.

Senator KENNEDY. Just on the West Nile?

Dr. GOODMAN. I am talking about a specific West Nile test.

Senator KENNEDY. West Nile, all right.

Dr. GOODMAN. Absolutely, sir.

Senator KENNEDY. Because the time is limited, the fact is that you are going to consider whether you are going to go ahead and mandate a test or not, and in what period of time, and how long will it take, estimate?

Dr. GOODMAN. OK. What we are aiming for is to work with the diagnostic and blood industry to rapidly assist and facilitate transfer of existing testing technology that is currently in place at CDC, other research labs, so that it can be done on broad scale if needed in a very rapid fashion.

In terms of the issue of mandate, there are two ways that FDA can assure that needed testing of blood is done. One is through regulation, normal comment and notice rulemaking, which, as you know, takes time. The other is we can issue a guidance for immediate implementation, which blood banks and the community have interpreted and followed as parts of our requirements for good manufacturing practices for blood. So as we continue to look at this evidence, we will issue guidance as and when needed, and I think we are behaving as if it will be needed.

And I would also say that the financial issues you raise are important ones. We do not make the diagnostic tests, and in a way, the industry needs to be able to see that there is a market in order to be incentivized to do this.

What I can report is based on a meeting we had with a number of key diagnostic firms and other parties last week, they are proceeding as if they perceive that there is a market and they are moving very rapidly to work with us and have testing available should we need it in a general way. But I support you.

Senator KENNEDY. My time has expired. I want to be clear. It seems to me that the evidence is sufficient that we ought to indicate a mandatory test and create the kind of climate and atmosphere where they are going to do what is necessary, and that is the financial investment to move ahead. It seems to me that we have the sufficient material. I thank the Chair.

Senator DURBIN. Thank you very much. Senator Gregg.

Senator GREGG. I do not want to pursue that discussion, but I have a lot of trouble mandating a test that does not exist. I think that the object is to get to a test that does exist and then determine whether or not to mandate it.

Senator KENNEDY. That is what it does, Senator. It only goes into effect when they get it. You create the business climate and the incentives to do it, and that is exactly the way it is done with this kind of a problem.

Senator GREGG. I am wondering whether the panel would comment on whether you should have spraying for the killing of mosquitoes. Do you consider this virus to be a significant enough threat that we should aggressively pursue in the various communities a policy of spraying?

Dr. GERBERDING. First of all, it is important to recognize that no pesticide is 100 percent safe, and so we do not want to use them if we do not have to use them.

The approach to controlling mosquitoes is really best done with an overall integrated approach, which starts with, as I said before, draining the standing water where the mosquitoes breed, wherever that is possible. In addition, using larvacides, which does not involve spraying and is a much safer, much less toxic form of mosquito control, can be done early in the year, often using organic materials that are safe for human health, is a very effective early season strategy that can attenuate the whole mosquito epidemic curve.

Spraying is really the last resort, and the technical assistance that CDC provides usually suggests that we not institute spraying programs until there are actually human cases in an area, because we try to deal with the problem through all other means first.

Senator GREGG. You mentioned this issue of DEET. I have got to revisit that, because I know in my region of the country, where there is a tremendous amount of hiking and woods activity, that for the last few years, there has been a very aggressive effort to not sell or use anti-mosquito lotions that include DEET because there was some perception that the DEET was a problem. It penetrated the skin and posed some significant health problems. But it is the position of the medical community that DEET is not a problem unless it is with a young child?

Dr. GERBERDING. That is the information we have available, but I will go back and——

Senator GREGG. No, that is fine. I just think we need to sort of clear the air on that, because there is a cottage industry out there saying, do not buy a product that has DEET in it, and it is quite aggressive, I can assure you, especially in the hiking community in New England.

If people have had a transfusion recently, what level of concern should they have, or if they have had some sort of major blood work, what level of concern should they have?

Dr. GOODMAN. I think, again, this is an issue that has to be kept in the broader perspective. We are taking this very seriously. We are very concerned by any transfusion-transmitted infection.

As I mentioned, there are several case reports which have been received by the Federal agencies in which blood transfusion is raised as a possibility for disease transmission, and one of these, the evidence is strong right now, we believe. So we have to take this seriously, although, again, as I mentioned, we have to take this in the context of 4.5 million people receiving blood in the United States a year.

So while we take this risk to the blood supply very seriously, and we are being very aggressive about it, for people for whom a blood transfusion is life saving or an organ transplant is life saving, the risk is likely to be much smaller than the potential benefit and people need to keep that in perspective. But in fairness, it is a rapidly evolving situation and we want people to be aware of the potential risk.

Senator GREGG. And what do you see as the time frame that you will have a screening test that could be generally accepted?

Dr. GOODMAN. I think it is an excellent question and I just wanted to also get back to a little bit of where Senator Kennedy's concern was coming from, that it would be very difficult for us through whatever regulatory process to say, you must perform a test that is not, in fact, currently available. What we are trying to do is everything we can to get it to the point where a test is available and we really are giving that message.

What we are hearing is that by doing several things, trying to work on technology transfer from existing tests—it is not as if things have not been developed which could be applied to this, but the issue is taking an existing test and potentially automating it and applying it to millions of samples. What we are hearing from partners in industry and the blood banks is that they are hopeful that they should be able to do this in time for the next major transmission season.

As I mentioned, there are some significant obstacles, but FDA also—we can help with this. We can allow use of these in a test situation before they are licensed to help provide additional public health protection. So certainly from FDA's point of view, this is a high priority. We will work with these companies. We will do whatever we can to help them get it out there. But in the end, we are not completely determinative——

Senator GREGG. Are we talking 6 months, a year, 2 years, 3 years?

Dr. GOODMAN. I think an optimistic version would be to have this available for next summer for the next major mosquito transmission season, at least for use in a study situation under investigational new drug status at FDA. If we can do it sooner than that, we would be delighted to see it used again in pilot tests, but I share your sense of urgency if this is needed. Thank you.

Senator GREGG. I appreciate the panel's commitment to this.

Senator DURBIN. Thanks, Senator Gregg.

Let me ask the panel, one of the most important things that we do here is to try to put things in perspective, and I think it is very important when we talk about issues of public health to put them in perspective. There is a tendency for us to rush to the disease du jour, and for the press and politicians to focus on that and to ask the American people with laser-like intensity to join us. And certainly on a daily basis, we pick up the newspaper, as Senator Warner did this morning, I hear from my home State, and Senator Landrieu, who will be back, hears about Louisiana constantly.

Dr. Fauci, when you put your poster up here about this challenge, you compared it to a flu pandemic and the AIDS epidemic. Put this in perspective for us so that we can understand what the public health threat is. The numbers from year to year are astounding in terms of growth. But in terms of the threat to Americans, give us your best analysis, and I will ask the other two doctors to join you.

Dr. FAUCI. Yes, and I think it is important, the point that you brought out. Certainly, quantitatively, when you look at the public health impact of the flu pandemic, which killed 25 million people, 750,000 in the United States; HIV/AIDS, 23 million dead, 40 million infected; I cannot imagine from knowing what we know about mosquito-borne diseases, how they spread, and the generally normal cyclic nature of flaviviruses—if you look at what happens with St. Louis encephalitis—it is extraordinarily unlikely that the impact of West Nile Virus would ever get onto the same radar screen as the two other diseases that I am talking about, flu and HIV/AIDS.

Having said that, this is a disease that we need to take seriously because it is not trivial. It is not going to wipe out scores of millions of people, but it is an evolving disease. This is the worst year that we have ever had. Hopefully, next year, we will see a downswing, the same way in the late 1970's with St. Louis encephalitis, when we had a disease that had 1,000-plus cases and then the next year it went right down.

But to say this is something trivial, I think would be far underestimating it. So not as bad as the major public health catastrophes that we had, but something we need to keep our eye on and be ready for the worst. That is my evaluation.

Senator DURBIN. In your business, in your profession, you measure the ebb and flow of an epidemic——

Dr. FAUCI. Right.

Senator DURBIN [continuing]. And you have just given us an example. Now, are we to surmise or conclude that based on what I think are fairly primitive responses to a mosquito-borne illness—insect repellant, fogging and spraying—that we can see a decline? Can we anticipate a decline in infections and deaths next year?

Dr. FAUCI. I think so. I think that there is certainly a possibility that with the preparation beforehand of mosquito control, alertness on the part of the public regarding the possibility, doing the kinds of things that Dr. Gerberding said, that it is quite likely that we will see a decrease. There is no guarantee.

The thing that we want to do is to do the public health measures that Dr. Gerberding spoke about. The blood protective mechanisms, regardless of what happens, forge ahead the way Senator Kennedy said about getting a diagnostic test for the blood, and at the same time have a vaccine available so that if in subsequent years we do not see a decline, if we see actually it continue to get worse and worse, then we will have a vaccine that we can vaccinate susceptible people, we will have a blood screening test, and the public health measures will be that much more experienced. So that is what my assessment would be.

Senator DURBIN. And let me ask the panel, for anyone who would like to respond to it now, and that is, if this is the type of virus that you have indicated, where if you have an immunity to another similar mosquito-borne illness, that it works against West Nile——

Dr. FAUCI. Partially.

Senator DURBIN. Partially. Let a liberal arts lawyer ask a doctor, why are we not immunizing, then, for one of these other possible illnesses with a safe vaccine, knowing that it will have a positive and prophylactic effect when it comes to the possibility of West Nile Virus infection?

Dr. FAUCI. There are two reasons for that. One, because the data in humans has not verified yet the data in animals. We are doing studies looking at—there are actually going to be studies that will be retrospectively going back, of people who have actually been vaccinated for yellow fever, what is the incidence if you do antibody tests to see if they have been infected with West Nile and/or gotten sick? So you can get scientific data. But the definitive proof that in humans it is protective does not have enough data to allow us to then say, based on animal models, we are going to go ahead and vaccinate.

The next issue is who to vaccinate. You certainly do not want to generally vaccinate the entire population, because the younger people really are at very little risk of serious disease. With some notable exceptions, there is very little risk.

Senator DURBIN. Is this similar to the flu vaccine, where we tell elderly Americans to be particularly attentive and stress the need for it?

Dr. FAUCI. Exactly.

Senator DURBIN. All right. Thank you.

Let me ask you, Dr. Gerberding, in terms of our response, we are talking about an added public health expense to a system that is already straining to keep up with all of the challenges, from sexually-transmitted diseases, immunizations for children, and others. As Senator Kennedy said, we just take it for granted that our public health system can absorb all these expenses. Now we are putting into it another challenge. Do we need to put more money into it, as well?

Dr. GERBERDING. The investments that we made this year were $29 million in the initial appropriation and then a supplement of $18 million that primarily went to the States that were the heaviest hit by the problem. That money was used to shore up surveillance and tracking of the disease in the birds and also to support the laboratories, but I think the system was stretched. Many of the laboratories report that they are at surge capacity. We have noted some delays in reporting the infection and getting the information back to us to track the epidemic. I think that we have done the best we can with the resources that we have, but the system is very stretched.

Senator DURBIN. Dr. Goodman, same question. Is this situation, the barriers of transferring the technology and new testing from the labs to the blood community, a question of money or personnel or time? What is it?

Dr. GOODMAN. I think it is more an issue at this point of technology, but I agree with your concern and Senator Kennedy's comment that the industry has to feel that there is a potential market here and be motivated by it. So I do think that is important. But as I said, again, the message that I am getting, at least informally and in recent meetings we have had, is that they are rising to the challenge and taking this very seriously and will move this along as quickly as possible.

Senator DURBIN. The last time I gave blood, there must have been 60 questions asked of me, maybe more.

Dr. GOODMAN. Right.

Senator DURBIN. Are there new questions being prepared for blood donors that really focus on West Nile Virus?

Dr. GOODMAN. Well, we are looking at this issue and working with the blood banking community closely. As I mentioned, the purpose of the alert back in August was the concern to prevent people with even mild symptoms of West Nile from donating blood. We are also working to be sure that people who subsequently develop an illness report it so that intervention can be made.

Some people have raised the issue, should we just be questioning donors about mosquito bites? Of course, the problem there is that one would exclude hundreds or thousands of donors for every one potentially protected. I think we simply need to know more about how much of this is out there to know how to best intervene.

Senator DURBIN. Thank you. Senator Warner, we have 5 or 6 minutes on the vote, but please, if you——

Senator WARNER. Why do you not go ahead and I will just stay.

Senator DURBIN. I am finished at this point in this round.

Senator WARNER. I was just going to take just a minute to return to my opening comments about what we might at this juncture in this problem advise the public who are following it, who are concerned for themselves, for their families. What steps should they take? Obviously, you spoke about the use of repellant, but I do not want to put the wonderful American tradition of the outdoor twilight barbecue out of our culture. What advice can you give us?

And second, most people are conscious when they are bitten by a mosquito. Sometimes you might not be aware when they make a pass at you, but what is the lapse time between the bite and the onset of the first symptoms?

Dr. GERBERDING. Let me address your first question. The population that I am the most concerned about are the elderly people, who are at the highest risk for the severe form of the disease. We have developed public service announcement and media campaigns to specifically target that population, in particular, advise them about the importance of, if they must go outside in the evenings or the early mornings, to use the insect repellant, but also just to wear an extra layer of clothing, and I know that is hard when the temperature is hot and it is humid outside, but to keep the skin covered and to do things like drain the water out of the water pots in the backyard. Most of the mosquitoes transmitting this virus live in the suburban backyard, and so the things you can do to eliminate their breeding ground can really help reduce the mosquito pool in the neighborhood.

Senator WARNER. Each of you who may have a little common sense advice.

Dr. FAUCI. Exactly. Just to reiterate what Dr. Gerberding said, it really is some fundamental, simple things that you can do, about warning everyone, particularly people who might be more susceptible to getting serious disease, and do some very simple things.

I go out in my own backyard—I live in Washington, DC, and every few days, you see something there that has collected water, be it a flower pot or an innertube or whatever that the children play with, and you just make sure every day you go out and turn it over and do not leave any standing water, because that really makes an impact.

Senator WARNER. I think they are obvious to us. What about the lapse time between your knowledge of being bitten and the likely onset of this problem?

Dr. GERBERDING. In general, the incubation period is usually just a few days, 2 to 4 days, but it can be longer. We have at least one patient with a flavivirus infection where we know the incubation period was 17 days. But most often, it is very short.

Senator WARNER. Any variation of that opinion?

Dr. FAUCI. No, that is about right, 3 to 15 days.

Senator WARNER. I thank the Chair for a very good hearing.

Senator DURBIN. Thanks, Senator Warner.

Let me ask, if I might, can we draw anything from the recent evidence or indication that this creates sometimes temporary polio-like symptoms? Is this a natural outgrowth of what we saw initially, what appeared to be encephalitis, or is this something new and alarming, or——

Dr. FAUCI. It is. It is new and alarming, because what we are seeing is that not only is this virus acting in an unusual way, as Dr. Gerberding pointed out, it is infecting virtually every known mosquito species. The mammalian, bird, and other range is much greater. Now we are starting to see clinical manifestations that if you open up a textbook and look under West Nile Virus and its manifestations, something like anterior horn cell, which is the cell that is infected to give you a polio-like syndrome, that is really rather novel for this. So we are concerned that the range of disease manifestations might be broader than what one would have originally thought when you think in terms of West Nile.

Senator DURBIN. Because our panel here has such great responsibilities and their time is very valuable, I am going to leave to vote and turn this over to Senator Hutchinson for questions and ask him if another Member arrives after he finishes, if he would pass the baton along. If not, we will just stand in recess until another Member does. Senator Hutchinson.

OPENING STATEMENT OF SENATOR HUTCHINSON

Senator HUTCHINSON. Thank you, Mr. Chairman. I apologize to the panel for having a conflict and only now arriving. I am not sure of everything that has been asked.

I represent the State of Arkansas, where we currently have 9 human cases of infection and 18 more are pending at the CDC for verification. Arkansas has also seen an unprecedented rate of infections among birds and horses. Positive birds have been found in 48 of the 75 counties in Arkansas. Our governor recently released $1 million in emergency funds for mosquito abatement at the local level, and this is in addition to almost $400,000 that was recently granted to the State by the Centers for Disease Control.

Now, as I understand, West Nile Virus has been common in parts of Africa, the Middle East, and Eastern Europe for many years. Because of the incidence in that part of the world, have there been any documented studies in these affected regions and countries about the transmission of the virus by means of blood transfusions or organ transplants?

Dr. GOODMAN. No. There were no documentations in the many areas where this disease has been epidemic or in previous years of infection in the United States of any infection spread by transfusion or organ transplantation. This was one of the factors which contributed to the assessment that while this was on the radar screen, the risk was likely to be low.

Senator HUTCHINSON. In the United States, how many cases have now been verified this year?

Dr. GOODMAN. Of West Nile?

Senator HUTCHINSON. West Nile.

Dr. GERBERDING. It is 1,947.

Senator HUTCHINSON. And the deaths have been?

Dr. GERBERDING. Ninety-four.

Senator HUTCHINSON. Ninety-four. Is that ratio consistent with what we see where the virus has existed for years and has been more common?

Dr. GERBERDING. In general, the mortality rate from the severe form of the infection, which is the brain or the meningitis form, is 10 percent, and that fatality rate has been the same for several years and is similar to the fatality rate observed in Europe. The ratio is not looking that way here because our total case count includes some of the much more milder forms of the illness, the so-called West Nile fever. So we do not have the right numerator and denominator together to give you the 10 percent.

Senator HUTCHINSON. Do they calculate the milder form at all, or are they only looking in other parts of the world at the more severe?

Dr. GERBERDING. In general, it is the more severe form of the illness that gets diagnosed accurately with the blood test, and so when we report cases, we are usually limited to the severe form, and that is where we calculate that 10 percent death rate.

Senator HUTCHINSON. Donor screening is one of the five parts of FDA's blood safety system. If most people infected with West Nile

Virus either show no symptoms or flu-like symptoms for just a few days, does donor screening become ineffective since a potential donor will not necessarily be conscious of the fact that they have the virus or they carry the virus?

Dr. GOODMAN. Yes, that is a real concern, that donor screening in terms of asking questions about how people are feeling, in terms of the medical exam for fever, as well as other measures we have been promoting, such as calling back if individuals develop illness and taking appropriate steps to protect blood safety, these will only deal with part of the problem if completely asymptomatic individuals can also transmit this by transfusion. So that is why as we are assessing the degree to which this is going on and a problem with the blood supply.

We are pushing on the development and technology transfer so that, if needed, there can be an actual blood test or donor screening test, because that would be really right now the only effective means of dealing with a problem, if it were a significant one, in the asymptomatic donors.

Senator HUTCHINSON. And we do not know right now how much of a problem it may be?

Dr. GOODMAN. Well, I would say we take any problem as a significant problem, and if you look at the fact, as you mention, that people can have the virus in their blood without having symptoms, we take that seriously. But right at this time, what we have is a few case reports under intensive investigation, some of which may represent this kind of transmission. But we are behaving as if they will show that this could occur and that we need to be prepared and potentially screen the blood.

One opportunity I would like to take, and perhaps Dr. Fauci or Dr. Gerberding would comment also, is that we were, or Dr. Fauci was asked earlier to put this in perspective with AIDS, which I think raises very important concerns and legitimate concerns when people hear about a disease that might be transmitted by blood, where this was such a problem for AIDS.

With West Nile Virus, there is a major important difference here, and that is that the currently available science would suggest that this virus is only in the blood for short periods of time in a donor. The donor then clears the infection. So it is not as if there is a reservoir of folks walking around chronically for months, years, lifetime with this in their blood. So that is an important distinction.

It does not mean that we do not need to take this seriously. And again, my point of view is, yes, we need a lot more information to know the degree of the risk, but while we are getting that information, we want to respond as if this risk were serious and significant and may require testing.

Senator HUTCHINSON. Let me just ask a kind of broad, open-ended question. Is there any tool or any additional authority that CDC should have in order to combat West Nile Virus?

Dr. GERBERDING. No. Our work in terms of controlling the mosquito component of the infection is based on cooperation with the State and local health officials. So the jurisdiction for making decisions about what kind of intervention program is appropriate are at the local level. We obviously are not a regulatory agency, but we do have, I think, very effective and supportive interactions with the public health community, and I think right now, our technical support is respected.

The training that we provide has been well received. An example of that is the fact that every laboratory, every public health laboratory in the United States has been trained by CDC to do the testing of the human cases, bird cases, and horse cases of West Nile. We provide the reagents and we have been able to document this year that that training has paid off, because the labs are doing a terrific job.

So we have the capacity to get the job done right and I do not think that our authority is the right limiting step in this. I think it is really simply the fact that this is an evolving epidemic and we do not know where it is going to go next.

Senator HUTCHINSON. Anybody else? Following up on your comments, do you have any reason to suspect that different strains of the West Nile might develop, and is the fact that some victims suffer paralysis while others do not have a sign that this could be a different strain?

Dr. GERBERDING. We have been working on characterizing the strains of the West Nile here in the United States since 1999 and comparing them to the strains that were involved in the outbreaks in the Middle East and Eastern Europe. What we have found is that, so far, all of the isolates that have been characterized in the United States are extremely similar, if not identical. So it looks like there is a single strain of West Nile evolving here.

Of course, the most recent isolates from these cases with polio-like illness and some of the other more unusual clinical syndromes are not fully characterized yet, so we look forward—that is one of our major research issues, is to do that strain characterization and look kind of at the strains from the standpoint of the illness that they create as well as the geography where they are located.

The strains that are here now are very similar to the strains that have been causing problems in Europe over the last 10 years, but not completely identical.

Senator HUTCHINSON. Thank you. My time is up. Senator Frist.

Senator FRIST. I apologize. We have been voting, so we may have covered some of these questions, but let me, while we have the opportunity, just go through some things real quickly.

In Canada and Mexico, what is happening in these areas; the maps kind of stop. Will the spread of West Nile Virus go further south, or what will be the natural history of it?

Dr. GERBERDING. There are cases reported in Canada, not surprisingly, given the bird migration patterns and the summer season there. We have one human case documented in Cayman Brac. That is the only documented case in the Caribbean so far, but the surveillance activities are just beginning to gear up in that part of the country and we are concerned about places such as Cuba or other areas in the Caribbean where we may not have the information about the mosquito infection or the bird infection the same way we do here, where——

Senator FRIST. Is there a potential for greater West Nile Virus spreading, place like Cuba, or as Senator Landrieu mentioned, Louisiana, the mosquitoes are going to transmit the virus year round. These areas could become a real haven for this virus, and then this is going to get a lot, lot worse. We do not have the controls; we cannot do the outreach; we cannot educate for the prevention. Obviously, you examine the history of malaria, the third biggest killer in the world, and its relationship to mosquitoes, to determine if we should be more concerned? What do we do?

Dr. GERBERDING. There is a concern. I think as this virus moves south through the Americas, we are alert to the fact that other mosquito-borne diseases are extremely effectively transmitted in Central America and South America. Dengue is one of those mosquito-borne diseases which is a close cousin of West Nile Virus infection.

What Dr. Fauci mentioned earlier, the mystery is, does infection with something like dengue give you a little bit of immunity to the West Nile Virus so that the population may be less at risk, or is it just another serious infection that we will have to add to the list? It is just too soon to tell.

Senator FRIST. Dr. Goodman and Dr. Fauci, the information on your slide that outlines the side effects of the smallpox vaccine and the low incidence of really severe infection; that information is based on data from earlier outbreaks. But, now that we have 900,000 people who are HIV-positive. We have my own profession of heart transplant in which thousands of transplants are being done every year. Additionally, about eight or nine million people who have cancer are either being treated or already immunocompromised. Could it be that those figures overall will be much higher, given today's population is very different than when most of that data was generated? You mentioned age, but if you could just paint that perspective for me.

Dr. FAUCI. The data of the 20 percent of people will develop mild symptoms and one to 150 to 200 are really very much in line with what we have seen from outbreaks in other countries. However, each year, one can then go back after the epidemic has essentially died down for the season and do sero-surveillance studies and get a feel for how many people in a given population were actually infected.

In fact, in New York, that very maneuver was accomplished, where they went back and looked at when you had the original 60 cases with X-number of deaths. You go back and in that Queens area of New York City that had the majority of cases, they found that about 2 to 3 percent of the entire population had been infected and they were able to then extrapolate that based on the identified clinically apparent cases to give you that ratio. We can easily do that by going back and doing retroactive sero-surveillance studies.

Senator FRIST. What are the three largest outbreaks in history? Did you all go through the history of West Nile before it entered the United States?

Dr. GERBERDING. We have not mentioned it in detail, other than to——

Senator FRIST. I think it is worth mentioning. If you had to look at the outbreaks, the first West Nile case appeared when? How large was the outbreak? What happened in the Middle East?

Dr. GERBERDING. The first case was documented in Uganda in 1937. I am not clear if that was associated with an outbreak or not. I think it was incidentally diagnosed. And then in the last 10 years, the largest outbreaks have been in Romania, Western Russia, and in Israel. A particularly noteworthy outbreak in Israel involved patients in a nursing home where there was a very high incidence of the encephalitis and the severe meningitis. So the largest outbreaks were clustered in that area of Europe and the Middle East.

Senator FRIST. Were there any long-term sequalae that appeared 5 years later, 10 years later, or 20 years later?

Dr. GERBERDING. We have studies ongoing now to follow the natural history of infected people, but it is too soon to say what the ultimate outcome would be. From the New York patients in 1999, many of those who survived the encephalitis remain with neurologic complications and fatigue syndromes and other serious disabilities.

Senator FRIST. Do these symptoms appear later or do they appear as a sequelae of the disease, the acute disease?

Dr. GERBERDING. Most of them had a continuum from having the illness and never regaining a full recovery.

Senator FRIST. Dr. Goodman, in organ transplantation, a single organ donor, who is generous and unselfish enough to having donated organs at the time of death, can transplant a heart, a lung, another lung, a pancreas, a kidney, obviously bone, tissue, eye, cornea, and help as many as 40 different people, one donor.

Dr. GOODMAN. Right.

Senator FRIST. And that is the beauty, and again, a plug for organ donation.

Given that one donor can affect 40 people, is it not incumbent upon us to have a crash course on how to screen that donor? What are we recommending to the transplant community? Right now, we screen donors routinely for HIV and for other infectious diseases. Have there been any policy recommendations for the transplant community, or are they being worked on?

Dr. GOODMAN. HRSA regulates the organ transplant testing, but we have been working closely with them and I think many of the same principles apply. I think you are right that this one instance of this organ transplant donor and the four recipients who developed infection is really the strongest case right now and is of great concern, and you are also right that in many cases, these people who choose to give this tremendous gift of organ donation may also donate tissues for a very diverse group of uses and that we are concerned about the potential for spread of the disease through those.

So to summarize that, I think the same push to get a practical, valid test which would allow us to screen blood is extremely and directly relevant to tissues and we support it for the same reason.

Senator FRIST. Do I have another minute?

Senator DURBIN. You certainly do.

Senator FRIST. I want to just clarify this testing business, if we can. Let us try to. Currently, there is a serologic test and a polymerase chain reaction (PCR), and yet there isn't a test for the blood supply.

Dr. GOODMAN. Let me try to be helpful on that.

Senator FRIST. My goal is to clear up for my colleagues and for people who are watching that when we say that there is not a commercially available test to do all this mass screening——

Dr. GOODMAN. Right.

Senator FRIST [continuing]. Which would be required to ensure the safety of our blood supply.

Dr. GOODMAN. Right.

Senator FRIST. Yet at the same time, we are making this diagnosis in all the people who have either been exposed or died from it. It is confusing to people that you have got a test for diagnosis, and yet there isn't a test for the blood supply. That being the case, how do we take the sort of testing that you can do and be able to make it broadly available so we can have these screens? What incentives—you say that is not your business to actually commercialize it, but is there something that we as policy makers can do to speed that process up?

Dr. GOODMAN. OK, a series of excellent questions. The first one, which is covered in written testimony but I can answer now here, too, is a real difficulty. Normally, the disease is diagnosed in a clinical laboratory or a State or the health department or the CDC through the presence in the blood of antibody to the infection, an early form of antibody called IGM. Now, that test is currently available and is being used to diagnose disease all over the United States.

Senator FRIST. Just so people understand, it is not the virus itself——

Dr. GOODMAN. Not the virus itself——

Senator FRIST [continuing]. It is the reaction to the virus. You are measuring what the body—the normal body response to the virus, so you are measuring that, not the virus.

Dr. GOODMAN. Exactly. This is measuring the host response in terms of producing antibodies to fight off the infection. Now, when a host does that, they rapidly appear to clear the virus from their blood.

So the problem from the issue of the blood supply, potentially, or the organ donor is that those individuals are unlikely to have antibodies in their blood. In fact, you could almost argue, if they did, they are probably at very low risk of transmitting the disease. So the same test that shows you that you might have West Nile Virus does not, in fact, does not correlate with showing you that you could transmit it to somebody.

And so in order to detect a risk for a blood or organ donor to transmit an infection to somebody else, you have to find direct evidence of the virus itself, not of the person's response to the virus because it is too soon. And as you mention, the technologies for doing that have predominately revolved around techniques which detect tiny amounts of the genes of the virus and amplify them to a level where they can be detectable. PCR, polymerase chain reaction, is one that is commonly utilized. There are other forms of nucleic acid amplification.

These tests are more complex, more technologically demanding, but on the positive side, we have succeeded in putting those kinds of tests in place to further reduce tremendously the risk of HIV and hepatitis C transmission in the blood to the order of less than one in a million or one in two million at this time. So I think we are optimistic that some of this technology is adaptable.

Senator DURBIN. Thanks, Senator Frist.

Dr. Goodman, I am sorry to hold the panel, but I want to follow up on that question, because earlier when we asked you about the blood supply, if I understood your answer correctly, you said we do not have a validated test at this point. Perhaps in a year, we might. We talked about the incentive for creating a mandate or a requirement for the test so that private industry, the private sector will respond with a test that we can use. Then you went on to say that you were considering new questions when it came to blood donors and you said if people exhibited flu-like symptoms, that might be an indicator of at least some concern or caution.

But I thought in just responding to Dr. Frist—Senator Frist and Dr. Frist at the same time—that you said if a person is asymptomatic, if they do not show any flu-like symptoms, they may still be carrying the West Nile virus, because the antibody is in their system.

Dr. GOODMAN. Right.

Senator DURBIN. So asking the question if they do not have any flu-like symptoms does not take us very far in terms of blood donors.

Dr. GOODMAN. Right. These are different components of steps to try to protect the American people from any risk here. One is to protect people through the donor questions and calling back if people have symptoms who may have infection and may manifest symptoms. But you are absolutely right. Another concern is the patients who do not have or never develop symptoms, and for those, a procedure such as testing the blood is what would be needed.

This also connects to Dr. Frist's question. But with respect to the incentive to the industry, etc., as I said, the message I am getting is that they are taking this seriously and proceeding full steam ahead. We are doing everything we can to push that level of preparedness and to do as a regulatory agency everything we can to facilitate that development. But in the end, the issue of the motivation and the performance of the industry is probably best addressed with them, but I have a positive perception so far.

Senator DURBIN. Thank you very much. The Senators who have arrived have said that they will save questions for the second panel.

I want to thank this panel and I want to make certain that what was said here is understood clearly and that I understood clearly, in that from Dr. Fauci, though we are not talking about a public health threat of the magnitude of the flu pandemic or AIDS disease, in your words, it is not trivial and must be taken seriously. You anticipate, and I hope you are right, a decline in infections and deaths next year from this problem. Is that fair?

Dr. FAUCI. It is possible that that would happen. There is certainly no guarantee. But if it acts like other flaviviruses have where there has been waxing and waning, we can expect, maybe not next year, that there will be a waning. It is unusual that you would see this, but we are prepared for that occurrence.

Senator DURBIN. And as far as a vaccine, a human vaccine, you say on an expedited schedule, 3 years is the likelihood of producing such a vaccine.

And Dr. Gerberding, what you have told us is local units of government and health agencies are going to need help in dealing with this mosquito-borne illness in terms of financial assistance. The $29 million this year has been helpful, but more will be needed in the future to deal with it, is that correct?

Dr. GERBERDING. Yes.

Senator DURBIN. Thank you very much. Dr. Goodman, Dr. Fauci, and Dr. Gerberding, thanks for joining us.

Senator DURBIN. Now we will move to the second panel. I will introduce them as they are being seated, in the interest of time for my colleagues.

Dr. Sidney Houff is here. He is the Professor and Chairman of Loyola University, Chicago's Department of Neurology. He will discuss the steps health care providers are taking to identify infections associated with the West Nile Virus, treat them, and educate the public about risk factors. In addition, he will outline how serious the threat is to humans, and the methods currently being used to treat the illness associated with the virus.

Dr. John Lumpkin, my friend and an outstanding public servant in the State of Illinois. We had a similar panel in Springfield in August. I am glad you are here today. Dr. Lumpkin is the Director of the Illinois Department of Public Health and will outline our State's current efforts, as I mentioned before, to control the spread of a virus which has hit us particularly hard.

Then we are going to have Dr. Fay Boozman, Director of the Arkansas Department of Health, to discuss additional challenges that State officials face when responding.

And we have one other witness, whom I will ask Senator Landrieu to introduce.

Senator LANDRIEU. The witness from Louisiana is Parish President Nickie Monica, who represents a parish right outside of New Orleans, actually between New Orleans and East Baton Rouge. Nickie has done an outstanding job in keeping the mosquito population down by putting in place a very effective eradication program that is both safe and effective.

We wanted him to share his insights, Mr. Chairman, because as much as we would like to have a vaccine, screening, and testing, I think our parishes and counties need some help with instituting appropriate kinds of spraying and pesticides programs that are so effective in preventing the spread of West Nile and the public feel safer. He is here to testify about that. Thank you, Nickie.

[The prepared statement of Senator Landrieu follows:]

PREPARED STATEMENT OF SENATOR LANDRIEU

I would like to begin by thanking the Chairmen and the Ranking Members of both of these committees for holding this very timely hearing. The recent outbreak of West Nile has demonstrated not only that we have learned a lot since our first experience with this deadly disease in 1999 but also that we have yet a lot more to learn. I am especially proud to be joined this morning by Nickie Monica, Parish President of St. John the Baptist Parish in Louisiana. Mr. Monica, and all of Louisiana local officials, have really been at the front lines in this war and have a great deal of insight to offer, especially in the area of mosquito abatement, a subject we are all too familiar with in my home state.

Mr. Chairman, as you know, the State of Louisiana, along with many other states, have for the past several months been under siege. The enemy is small, but powerful, and great in number. Hard to detect, they sneak up on you and with one attack, they can change your life forever, because they carry with them a deadly weapon to which we have little defense. To date, 11 Louisianans have lost their lives in our war against mosquitoes and the West Nile Virus that they carry and 261 more have been made ill, In Baton Rouge, our state capital, 42 people have been reported to be infected with the disease and three have died. Only Illinois, with 473 human cases and 25 deaths, has experienced more casualties from the virus than Louisiana.

In 2000, the Governmental Affairs Committee, under the direction of my esteemed colleague Senator Lieberman, did a study of our Nation's response to the first recorded outbreak of West Nile in the Western Hemisphere. While their ultimate conclusion was that local, state and federal officials had acted with the speed and skill necessary to control the outbreak, doing so required that they overcome a series of barriers that inhibited them in many ways. Our recent experience in Louisiana has demonstrated that many of these barriers still remain. I will touch on three remaining barriers here this morning.

Throughout the history of Louisiana, spraying for mosquitoes and dredging the water they breed in has been a common occurrence. Until now, however, it was done because mosquitoes were pests and they could carry deadly germs. Now, our state and local officials are spraying around the clock in a desperate race to control the worst outbreak of West Nile the Western hemisphere has ever seen. There is no specific treatment for West Nile, nor a vaccine. The most effective way to protect our citizens against this deadly virus is to stop it before it happens.

I recently introduced legislation, along with members of my delegation, that asks for federal assistance for states to "M.A.S.H." out this predator and stop the spread of this disease. I think that is clear that there is an urgent need for this bill to become law. If passed, it can have an immediate effect in saving on the lives of people in my state and throughout the nation. One might think that funding of this type is already available, but it is not. In fact, the $3.4 million that Louisiana received from the CDC this August was specifically directed at other purposes such as treatment, public awareness campaigns and testing. What's more, this funding is given from the federal to the state government and is often inadequate to get to down to the local level, where it is arguably needed the most.

I want to be clear, however, that this legislation is not an effort to supplant state's responsibility in this area, but to supplement it. Our state has and will continue to dedicate a great deal of state and local resources toward "Fighting the Bite." On September 5, 2002, the State of Louisiana began distributing $3.4 million in state funds to support the local governments in their efforts to combat West Nile. The Department of Health and Hospitals is spending over $200,000 on a public education campaign asking people to do their share to avoid leaving standing water and other mosquito havens. Two-thirds of Louisiana's population is covered by an active mosquito control program and those without mosquito control programs are using spray trucks provided by the Louisiana Department of Agriculture and Forestry.

The second barrier is somewhat related to the first. Our Nation's first experience with the West Nile Virus taught us that effective treatment and prevention of this deadly disease requires coordination among the many federal agencies with expertise and jurisdiction in outbreaks of this kind. The formation of a West Nile Virus Coordinating Committee, chaired by the CDC and composed of representatives from USDA, the United States Geological Survey's National Wildlife Health Center, the Environmental Protection Agency, FEMA and the U.S. Defense Department was a first step in this direction. These efforts must be strengthened and pushed beyond just the walls of the Coordinating Committee. An effective response to this disease not only requires the advice, but the resources and personnel, that can be balled upon by all of the agencies represented on the Coordinating Committee. I urge this committee to explore ways that we can improve the coordination of these federal agencies and their sate and local counterparts.

Finally, as the committee recognized in 2000, the United States public and animal health communities remain divided culturally and organizationally. This divide continues to raise serious public health concerns, especially in prevention and treatment of diseases that are transmitted from animals to humans, such as West Nile. Dr. Maxwell Lea, Louisiana's state veterinarian, has reported to us that well over one hundred horses are confirmed to have died from the disease. He also reports that several times this many deaths have gone unreported. Often times the greatest number of livestock deaths coincided with the level of human incidence. I would suggest that we explore ways to bridge this divide so we can stop the spread of the disease before it results in death to humans or the livestock they depend on.

Mr. Chairman, thank you again for the opportunity to be here and to participate in this hearing. I am very proud to represent the citizens of the Great State of Louisiana who, I think you will agree, have done a tremendous job under extreme pressure. On behalf of them, I thank you for your continued work in this area.

Senator DURBIN. Thanks, Senator Landrieu.

At this point, under the rules of the Senate Governmental Affairs Committee, I will ask you all to please rise for the oath.

Do you solemnly swear the testimony you are about to give is the truth, the whole truth, and nothing but the truth, so help you, God?

Dr. HOUFF. I do.

Dr. LUMPKIN. I do.

Mr. MONICA. I do.

Dr. BOOZMAN. I do.

Senator DURBIN. Let the record indicate that the witnesses have answered in the affirmative.

I am sorry, Senator Hutchinson. I thought you had left, but would you like to say a word about Dr. Boozman before they give their testimony?

Senator HUTCHINSON. Mr. Chairman, I would only rarely correct you, but his name is pronounced Boozman.

Senator DURBIN. Boozman, I am sorry.

Senator HUTCHINSON. Dr. Boozman is our Director of the State Department of Health in Arkansas, is doing an outstanding job, and is a very dear friend of mine and we are glad to have him on our panel today. Thank you, Mr. Chairman.

Senator DURBIN. Thank you.

Dr. Houff, would you like to be the first to testify?

TESTIMONY OF SIDNEY ANDREW HOUFF, M.D., PH.D.,[1] PROFESSOR AND CHAIRMAN, DEPARTMENT OF NEUROLOGY, AND DIRECTOR, NEUROSCIENCE AND AGING INSTITUTE, LOYOLA UNIVERSITY MEDICAL CENTER, MAYWOOD, ILLINOIS

Dr. HOUFF. Mr. Chairman, Members of the Committee, I want to thank you very much for the opportunity to be here today. I am not only the Professor and Chair of Neurology at Loyola University, but I would like to tell you that I am the Chair of the Steering Committee for the Conservation Medicine Center of Chicago and the Director of the Neuroscience and Aging Institute, and I think those are important because the Conservation Medicine Center is a collaborative effort between Loyola University, the Brookfield Zoo, and the University of Illinois, bringing a consortium of veterinarians, physicians, and so forth together addressing this sort of problem.

I would like to divide my testimony up into two aspects. One, I would like to give you a clinical impression of what these patients are like. I have had the privilege and the honor of taking care of them, and give you some idea of what we are facing in the human area, and then speak to you as a neurovirologist and someone responsible for designing and implementing studies of these kinds of illnesses.

First, I would like to let you know that us in the medical community are privileged and pleased with the response of the CDC and State health departments. The response has been tremendous. It has been very informative and efficacious for us as physicians taking care of these patients, and I think that the congratulations and

---

[1] The prepared statement of Dr. Houff appears in the Appendix on page 64.

debt of the medical community to these groups has been well founded.

As far as the clinical aspects of this disease, it is my opinion we have seen some changes in the clinical manifestations of this disorder. In the past, the neurological complications have been mainly meningeal encephalitis, that is an inflammation of the brain, and the meninges, the covering of the brain, with very little seen in what we call focal neurologic deficits, that is, the deficits that cause paralysis or those sorts of things.

In the beginning in 1999, we did see what was called Guillain-Barre-like illness, where people became profoundly weak with muscle pain. But in this episode, or this epizootic, what we have noticed is focal neurologic deficits have been more common. Now, whether that is going to hold up true at the end of the epidemic when we look at all the cases, I do not know. But certainly in our experience in Chicago, that has been a prominent finding, that we have begun to see patients with optic nerve disease and blindness, anterior horn cell disease and paralysis, Parkinson's-like syndromes, and so forth during the acute illness. So that really strikes to us as a change in the clinical picture may be occurring as this epidemic evolves over the years.

As far as treatment goes, as you know, it is very limited. We only have supportive therapy at the present time. We use steroids to reduce brain swelling, we use seizure medications to prevent seizures, and we support the patients. Unfortunately, as you know, that is not always possible to do and we have had deaths, both at Loyola and other institutions in Chicago.

As far as treatment, you have heard from Dr. Fauci what lays on the future. One of the things that I would emphasize is the possibility of using immunoglobulin therapy, gammaglobulin therapy, and antibody therapy for this. We do know in neurological diseases in the past we have been successful with that. For instance, in enterovirus like polio, we have been able to treat patients who have low gammaglobulin levels successfully with this type of therapy.

And in Israel, there is at least one case that I am aware of that has been treated with serum containing high antibodies to West Nile Virus and the patient survived. Whether that was a direct effect or not, I do not know. But certainly, that is something that one could address quickly and bring to the forefront in a short period of time as a way to address a possible illness.

Switching gears and talking about what we do not know about West Nile Virus and what I think would be a reasonable approach in the future, I think that Illinois has a very interesting history that may be quite illuminating if we approach it correctly. As you know, Illinois was faced with the St. Louis encephalitis virus epidemic in the 1970's which was quite severe, and as you heard earlier, the St. Louis encephalitis virus and West Nile Virus are both filioviruses.

So one of the questions I think that it behooves us to address in the future is what is different here? What in the enzootic, what animal species, what avian species are infected, what mosquito species are infected, and why in this environment do we face so many animal cases and so many human cases? I think that Illinois offers us an opportunity to address those issues. With that in mind, the

Conservation Medicine Center of Chicago is now looking into designing studies to address those issues, both in the animal population, the insect population, and in the human population.

Finally, I would like to address surveillance because I think this epidemic illustrates what we are up against. We have done a fine job at identifying things and identifying West Nile Virus and plotting its development, but one of the things we have done over the years is close many of the surveillance centers around the world. As jet travel and human travel between countries has increased, we have decreased our surveillance efforts around the world, and I would encourage people who have the opportunity and the ability to think about reopening those to address emerging infections.

Senator DURBIN. Excuse me, Doctor. Could you be specific? When you say surveillance efforts, what are you talking about?

Dr. HOUFF. Yes, sir. I will be glad to, Senator Durbin. The Rockefeller Institute, for instance, has centers around the world that monitored arbovirus infections, infections that were transmitted by insects and so forth, and those were closed as the years went by and they are not available anymore. So what we do not know is how are these viruses circulating in nature in other areas.

One of the questions that came earlier this morning was do we know whether West Nile Virus circulates in the United States in animal populations and humans as it does in Europe and the Middle East, and although we think we do, the actual studies that we need to do to address those issues specifically have not been done and need to be done. If you look at the epidemic in Israel, for instance, and the United States, we have had high avian die-offs in both. The Romanian epidemic was not associated with that, nor were any other West Nile Virus infections that I know of. So these surveillance centers, I think, are very critical for the future.

Senator DURBIN. Thank you very much, Dr. Houff.

Dr. HOUFF. Thank you, sir.

Senator DURBIN. Dr. Lumpkin.

TESTIMONY OF JOHN R. LUMPKIN, M.D.,[1] DIRECTOR, ILLINOIS DEPARTMENT OF PUBLIC HEALTH, SPRINGFIELD, ILLINOIS

Dr. LUMPKIN. Thank you, Mr. Chairman, and thank you for the opportunity, and the Members of the Committee, to speak and talk a little bit about our experience in Illinois.

Illinois, as you know, is one of the most severely impacted States in the Nation. As of today, we will be reporting in the neighborhood of 520 cases. There was at least one additional death we will be reporting today, which will bring our total up to 28. This obviously has had a tremendous impact and it is not a trivial outbreak.

Our experience in Illinois began last year when we had our first case of birds that was found to be positive for West Nile. We have had an avian surveillance system that has been in place. It has been in place since 1976. We, on average, collect about 5,000 birds. We trap them live, we draw blood, and we have been testing since that time. That surveillance system, as well as the collection of birds and other animals, gave us a heads up that we were going to have problems.

---

[1] The prepared statement of Dr. Lumpkin appears in the Appendix on page 67.

We have had in place plans to begin to address West Nile through support from the Centers for Disease Control. Our first plan was put in place in May 2001, prior to any cases in Illinois, and then we developed a task force under the direction of the governor of State agencies that began to put our plans in place for this spring.

Our first case amongst birds was found in May. We saw an outbreak that really moved fairly slow until mid-July, in which case there was an explosive outbreak amongst the birds. In many neighborhoods, particularly in the Chicago area, it has been called the "silent summer" because birds have not been heard in many communities. There really has been a dramatic impact upon the bird population.

In response to this and with the subsequent human cases, we began to use State resources. We had made grants to local health departments to develop plans prior to the human cases, but afterwards, $3 million of State funding were made available. This has created certain problems for us, because as we have looked at how to address the resources that we have available, and with the State, like many other States, having severe budget restrictions, we have essentially had to use money that currently would be available to local health departments to do food inspections, infectious disease control, inspections of water and sewage systems, and so we have had to dip into that fund and spend money that we really do not have in order to respond to the West Nile.

We are currently engaged in activity. This $3 million has been granted out to counties throughout the State that have had human cases. We have been focusing on doing larvaciding as well as integrated mosquito control. This integrated control has had an impact. We believe that our outbreak obviously would have been much worse had we not been able to do this sort of response.

I would like to talk about one issue that was raised and one that is a concern. We have a number of things in place in Illinois, surveillance and our response plan, basically because we responded to an outbreak in 1975. Since that time, many of the mosquito abatement districts at the local level had seen significant reductions in resources. We as a Nation and many communities tend to forget the lessons that we have learned from the past, and as such, it became incumbent upon the State to make resources available to local communities when those communities exhausted the resources that were available at the local level.

But an important question, I think, has to be raised. First, do we really understand this disease and are we conducting studies in all the ways that we should? The first panel talked about research that is going on in humans. I wonder whether or not we are doing adequate research among the avian population, the major reservoir. Do we fully understand this? What will be the pattern? I do not think the answer will be in people. I think the answer will be in birds. What is their experience? Why are we seeing such a large bird die-off?

The second is that when you look at the cases in Illinois, three-quarters of the cases in Illinois are in Cook County. Over half of those cases are in two distinct locations, the exact same locations that we had a major number of cases in 1975 in our St. Louis encephalitis outbreak.

Senator DURBIN. Which locations are those?

Dr. LUMPKIN. That is the Southwest side, mainly focused around the Oak Lawn area, Evergreen Park, Beverly, Morgan Park, that area, and on the North side, sort of focused around Skokie, dipping into the city in that area.

I think that there is reason to do intensive study of those communities to find out what in particular is about the bird population and the mosquito population that leads to the recurrence of this particular outbreak so severe in a virus that is very similar to St. Louis encephalitis. I think we missed an opportunity to do that research in 1975 and we should not miss that opportunity to do that research this year because of the severity of the outbreak.

We are looking for assistance from the Federal Government. I think we have had a fair, a good bit of assistance in the past, but we need to have additional research to better handle—give us the kind of tools. Some of the tools that we need, for instance, are how we conduct our bird surveillance. We collect blood samples from wild birds. I do not think we have adequate reagents to be able to test them as a very early warning system to be able to determine whether or not West Nile Virus exists in those bird populations. Understanding more about the biology of West Nile in the bird population is worth additional research, and as well as resources should be made available to the States and communities to better respond. Thank you.

Senator DURBIN. Thanks a lot. Mr. Monica, thank you for joining us.

TESTIMONY OF NICKIE MONICA,[1] PARISH PRESIDENT, ST. JOHN THE BAPTIST PARISH, LaPLACE, LOUISIANA

Mr. MONICA. Mr. Chairman, Members of the Committee, I am Nickie Monica, Parish President of St. John the Baptist Parish, and resident of the suburb of the New Orleans metropolitan area. St. John's population is near 50,000 residents and is one of the fastest growing areas in the State of Louisiana. St. John is located on the Mississippi River, which has a substantial industrial job base that has brought significant economic development and higher than average wages to our area.

It is indeed a pleasure to appear before your Subcommittee to shed some light on the growing local problem that has national implications. Just a short time ago, mosquitoes, like many other insects, were just another nuisance that interrupted the outdoor life of our residents. Unfortunately, it has now been thrust into the national media because it has become a serious health hazard, with devastating consequences to many families around this country, including those in my State of Louisiana.

Fortunately, Mr. Chairman, St. John Parish has not yet experienced a human fatality, something I believe is due to our proactive measures to combat this growing public menace. However, if a more prominent effort is not put forth, I am fearful that it is just a matter of time before tragedy strikes home.

---

[1] The prepared statement of Mr. Monica appears in the Appendix on page 69.

St. John the Baptist Parish initiated its own regimented mosquito control program over a decade ago. That was an added quality of life issue for our residents. This program is run by professional and licensed entomologists who are experienced in the field of surveillance and treatment. Our spraying and treatment program experienced no problems until the West Nile Virus began approaching Louisiana from the East Coast States. We immediately allocated 30 percent more funding to the spraying program without additional surveillance. We also began a public awareness campaign to encourage residents to minimize the threat of larvae hatchings around homes and businesses. Additionally, the Louisiana Department of Health and Hospitals initiated statewide public service announcements reminding all residents to be vigilant and lessen the threat of infection. It is my opinion this has been effective in itself.

Even though St. John the Baptist Parish has an adequate control program in place, our financial ability to continue to fight over a sustained period of time is practically exhausted. We all know this problem is not going away. The question is how best to fight and fund an effective program. The fact that parishes and cities that do have a program also have West Nile Virus, that is of great concern.

Mr. Chairman, I know my own parish and State best and have thoughts on how to provide a remedy to abate danger. We now have to look to the experts to tell us what is best, the best protocol that could be implemented statewide. It is definitely more than a local program. It is a national and State health concern, and the Federal Government does need to play a major role in fighting and funding. Of course, any Federal program must be consistent statewide in order to maximize abatement efforts.

Mr. Chairman, I also want to thank the Louisiana Congressional delegation and the U.S. Congress for their efforts to assist Louisiana and the rest of the affected areas of our country in this effort. For example, further Federal assistance should immediately begin to provide rapid processing of bird and mosquito specimens submitted for virus testing, and that would be made possible by the Mosquito Abatement for Safety and Health Act, S. 2935, as introduced by Senators Breaux and Landrieu. The legislation could allow State and local governments to react more rapidly by providing funding to existing programs and States.

Too much time has been lost in reporting results that could further direct control efforts. The point of surveillance is to detect the virus before it spreads to the human population. When weeks are required to report results, the advantage of an early warning system is lost. Consequently, immediate preparation and funding are needed to allow State laboratories to continue testing dead birds submitted by citizens even after the virus activity has been detected in a particular parish or county. The additional data is vital in determining the exact location of the virus, which, in turn, allows more direct assignment of abatement resources.

The Congress should also continue emergency funding for expanded surveillance, for testing, and for State laboratories, which will play a role in early detection of the virus. My parish needs assurances that emergency supplemental funds will be made available for additional mosquito control efforts should West Nile or any other mosquito-borne disease require response beyond our local capabilities. This becomes particularly important when disease is coupled with storms or manmade catastrophes that stretch available resources beyond their limits.

Mr. Chairman and Members of the Committee, this concludes my testimony. It was indeed a pleasure to be able to convey my thoughts on an important issue and a growing national health problem that will require a unified effort. I want to thank each of you for your participation and I will be available to answer any questions. Thank you, Mr. Chairman.

Senator DURBIN. Thanks, Mr. Monica. Dr. Boozman.

TESTIMONY OF FAY W. BOOZMAN, M.D., M.P.H.,[1] DIRECTOR, ARKANSAS DEPARTMENT OF HEALTH

Dr. BOOZMAN. Thank you, Mr. Chairman and Committee. I appreciate the opportunity to share with you. I have been very appreciative of the experts that have been testifying to you because they are the same experts we depend upon to guide us. But I feel like the report I am going to give you is somewhat of a blue collar report in the sense that while vaccines are being developed and these very important questions that you have been asking are being looked at, we are faced on a daily basis with people contracting this disease and a need to deal with it.

I want to thank our partners at the CDC. They have been outstanding in giving us funding and being as flexible with that funding as they can be and helping us to meet this crisis. They have been excellent in helping with our surveillance, our laboratory, and the other things, and I think that money that you have already spent was wisely spent and has done an awful lot.

There has been a lot of talk in the testimony about next year, and I certainly do not speak from any scientific perspective. I am just looking at what has been happening. This has gone down the East Coast. It is coming from the North. As a State health officer, I have to think we are going to have a bad year next year. The year we are having this year is very much like the year Louisiana had last year and the disease burden is just growing. The virus burden is clearly growing. Last year, we had four birds. This year, we are up in the hundreds of birds.

And so I feel like that we have got to build on the knowledge we have. As new knowledge is being developed, we have got to build on the knowledge we have. We know that larvaciding works. We know that getting rid of standing water and places where the mosquitoes can breed, education in those areas works.

Recently in Pine Bluff, Arkansas, which is our focal area, where we have the most cases, they had a community clean-up and the county judge told me that they did not pick up a single tire in that county that did not have growing mosquito larvae in it when they picked it up. So there are things that can be done that we need to be doing right now that we know needs to be done while we work out some of these very important questions.

In Arkansas, we estimate that a good comprehensive, integrated program of education, larvacide, and then in those areas where we

---

[1] The prepared statement of Dr. Boozman appears in the Appendix on page 70.

have significant human cases, adulticide, would cost in the neighborhood of about $5 million. This year——

Senator DURBIN. Excuse me, Doctor. You used the term adulticide?

Dr. BOOZMAN. Yes, of the mosquitoes, the adult mosquitoes, the spraying.

This year, our governor released out of his emergency fund $1 million, which we specifically just used for larvaciding. Larvaciding, I think, is the most efficient and most cost effective and safest in terms of a way to help control the mosquito population.

I think we certainly need to continue the surveillance activities that have already started. As Senator Frist mentioned in some of his questions earlier, there is an awful lot of overlap as we prepare for this with our preparations for bioterrorism. In fact, as we have responded to the West Nile, through our communications, through the many different things we have done, I think it has made us much better able to respond to a bioterrorist event. I think it is money that is actually having a good dual purpose. As our surveillance gets better for West Nile, it gets better for everything else, also.

I think we have clearly seen that we have got to continue to invest in the capacity of our public health laboratories. We saw it with anthrax and it has just been amplified with this, that we do not have the capabilities at the State level right now. There has not been much investment in public health laboratories for many years, and as a result of that, we need to continue to increase their capacities.

So in conclusion, Mr. Chairman, I think we must continue the funding that has been going on in surveillance, the additional funding we got that allowed us for the education. But I think there has got to be some additional funding for vector control of these mosquitoes. And also, though we have had some funding, I think there has to be a continued emphasis on getting our public health laboratories into shape. Thank you, sir.

Senator DURBIN. Thanks, Dr. Boozman.

Let me first ask of Dr. Lumpkin, you have focused on two areas in the Chicago area which may be beyond our parochial interest, since we are from the same State, and you indicated that the incidence of St. Louis encephalitis in these same two areas where you are seeing the prevalence now of West Nile Virus infection is worthy of investigation. Could you follow up a little bit on the 1975 that you referred to, was there a similar situation with the death of the bird population, the avian population?

Dr. LUMPKIN. I am not aware that there was a similar death of the avian population, but I think we heard earlier testimony there were roughly 1,000 or more cases of St. Louis encephalitis that year. Almost 600 of those were in Illinois, and there were 47 deaths. So it was the most intense experience of St. Louis encephalitis.

Senator DURBIN. Mosquito-borne?

Dr. LUMPKIN. Mosquito-borne, intensified in birds. The difference between West Nile and St. Louis encephalitis is the West Nile Virus replicates much more rapidly than St. Louis encephalitis. So many of the conditions between West Nile and St. Louis encephalitis are very similar. So if we had an intense experience in 1975, why? And if we have the same intense experience with a similar kind of vector-borne, same mosquitoes and birds, why again?

What we learned with basic epidemiology is you identify the population that appears to be most at risk and you study them intensely to see if you can learn the kind of lessons that then become applicable to the general population, and we believe that would be the case in the areas that are intensely involved in Illinois.

Senator DURBIN. I think that is worth following up, not just for our own protection, but perhaps for the lessons learned for other parts of the country.

I just looked. Back in July, we announced some money through the Department of Agriculture for the State of Illinois, $750,000 to deal with this. At the time, I noted in my press release, I made a point that there had not been a case of human infection as of July 26 of this year, and here we are with, I believe, hundreds of cases of infections, including an incident with a young intern on my staff who went down to the Illinois State Fair in Springfield, came home not feeling well, and we thought she had meningitis. That was the first diagnosis when she—she is fortunately a young, healthy woman and went to the hospital for 2 or 3 days, came back, felt better, recovered. Two weeks later, they told her she was a victim of West Nile Virus which she did not realize. But now, in that short span of time, there have been 27 or 28 fatalities in our State.

Let me ask you the question which continues to come to mind, and I would like Mr. Monica or perhaps others to respond to it. What is the trade-off here? When we start using larvacides, insecticides, adulticides, what is the downside, if there is any? Is there a danger associated with spraying these chemicals and the impact it might have on public health or the public water supply as opposed to the danger of West Nile Virus? How do we balance these and come to the right conclusion?

Dr. LUMPKIN. Well, West Nile Virus, getting West Nile Virus comes down to the numbers. In areas where there have been an intense experience with West Nile, roughly one out of 200 mosquitoes will carry West Nile Virus. And for those who are bitten, one out of 150 will get the severe form. So those odds are about one to 30,000 mosquito bites. The best mosquito abatement can reduce the mosquito population by 50 percent.

Senator DURBIN. Fifty?

Dr. LUMPKIN. Fifty percent. So you now reduce the risk because you are reducing the number of mosquito bites. So when you start to see that you are having transmission, you need to use all your tools. The first tool is larvaciding. You kill them. You prevent them from hatching into adults so they cannot go around and bite the birds and bite people. Once you begin to have intense experience, as we have done in these two areas, then we use adult spraying, so the combination of the two.

We do not support nor do we fund adult spraying only. Adult spraying will only have a short-term effect. It will last a couple of days. Larvaciding lasts for weeks.

Senator DURBIN. But I am asking you, is there a public health risk to the larvacide and the adulticide and other forms of mosquito control?

Dr. LUMPKIN. Yes. The risk to larvaciding is very minimal. It is a fairly specific chemical that is targeted to mosquitoes. The risk for adult spraying, any kind of spraying, because of particulate matter, may impact someone who has sensitivity to the chemicals. But the studies that were done in 1999 in New York indicated that the risk from West Nile was greater than the risk from the chemicals. And so I think we get to the point when we begin to see human cases that the public health equation says we take the risk for the better good and we give public warning so people who may have those sensitivities stay indoors.

Senator DURBIN. In Illinois, we have focused on and made certain that there is spraying in the two target areas that you mentioned, the Skokie area as well as the Oak Lawn-Beverly-Evergreen Park area?

Dr. LUMPKIN. That is correct, and then there is focused spraying depending upon bird surveillance and mosquito surveillance around the State.

Senator DURBIN. Thank you.

Mr. MONICA. Mr. Chairman, I have a comment.

Senator DURBIN. Certainly. Mr. Monica.

Mr. MONICA. I think it is important to have a comprehensive mosquito control program in place because, No. 1, you larvacide, No. 2, our program, we set traps and we monitor the traps and we collect the adult mosquitos and that is to determine our spraying. But during dry periods, sometimes there is no need to spray. So I think it is really important that we come with a unified program, because mosquitoes and infected birds do not know parish lines, county lines, or State lines. So I think it is important that we develop a plan and unify a plan and attack this problem. But having a comprehensive program in place, I think, is what benefitted St. John Parish to this point.

Senator DURBIN. Thank you. I have another question of Dr. Houff, but I want to let my colleague, Senator Frist, ask at this point.

Senator FRIST. Thank you, Mr. Chairman.

Dr. Houff, I stepped out while your oral presentation was made. Could you comment on what we were talking about earlier in terms of the immunosuppressed patient or the immunocompromised patient in any way, whether it is from age or it is from immunosuppressants for transplantation or cancer therapy. Does this population worry you more than the non-immunosuppressed population in terms of manifestation or ease of treatment?

Dr. HOUFF. Yes, sir, it does. I think that is an excellent point. One of the things we do not know is what is the host immune response? What is the patient's immune response? Is it just cellular immunity, hemo immunity, or the combination of the two? It is likely the combination of the two.

We have seen West Nile in heart transplant patients, two that I am aware of, and that population does worry me considerably because, as you know, when those kinds of individuals get infected, any kind of therapy you have is more limited. We know that from a lot of different infectious diseases. Once the patient is immuno-suppressed, the antiviral therapies we have, the interferons, what-ever we have, antibiotics, are not as efficacious. And so this popu-lation, which is rising—I think you made that point earlier today, the population of immunosuppressed patients rising with an in-creasing number of birds dead and mosquitoes dead in urban popu-lations, where a lot of this disease and a lot of transplants and so forth is done, is quite concerning.

Senator FRIST. Have we talked about contagiousness of this virus today? I am not sure if we brought it up, but did you bring it up at all?

Dr. HOUFF. I did not bring it up.

Senator FRIST. You might just comment on the risk for person-to-person transmission. When we are talking the bioterror agents, it is real clear. Anthrax, we finally made it clear that it is not a contagious microorganism. Smallpox is. Please comment on the ability to transmit West Nile from person-to-person because I think the potential of this whole hearing is to outline the impact in peo-ple's lives with the first panel and, in the second panel, to outline our response and whether we are behind the curve. But, if you could just comment on that again for our edification.

Dr. HOUFF. Besides the discussions about blood and organ trans-plants, I know of no human-to-human transmission of this agent. As a caveat to that, I think one of the things that has not been dis-cussed this morning is the spill-over into other mammals. The Illi-nois public health has reported squirrels and dogs. That has been reported in the past. There have been a lot of mammals reported in the past in some of these epidemics around the world.

The critical factor is, they appear to not get enough virus in the blood to be infectious for mosquitoes. But we do know that lemurs in Madagascar, for instance, can transmit West Nile to mosquitoes in nature, and there are some reptile species that can transmit the virus to mosquitoes.

And so I think one of the emphases that we should do is look at what are the mammal populations that has been infected during this episode and what are the titers of virus in those animals, be-cause I think that may be a critical epidemiological issue.

Senator FRIST. I think it is important, and we have not talked much about it today, that science really is being developed broadly. I was at the Smithsonian Institution yesterday talking to a range of people, and there is a whole cadre of people working on trans-mission—experts in mosquitoes. This whole issue of its spread by migratory birds is rather complex, including determining what type of birds which can spread the virus.

One of the Smithsonian researchers there, John Rappole, who is at the CRC, Conservation Research Center, had written an article in the *Journal of Applied Microbiology*. In that article, he stated that the migratory birds historically have not been a good can-didate for transmission because the disease had been moving much slower than expected. However, the resident species might be a much better carrier.

I think it is going to be important as we look at spread and its potential spread, we need to expand the science around species and species transmission.

44

Dr. LUMPKIN. In addition, I think there is one other factor. The evidence related to the transplantation-related cases and the transfusion-related cases brings up the whole issue of people who are hunters. There is no evidence of transmission by people normally in contact with animals, but certainly there is reason to believe that it is possible to have transmission if you are, in fact, in contact with blood from an animal that has been recently killed. So the recommendations that we have made and continue to make for hunters, that they be careful when they are dressing down animals, for West Nile and other diseases, still applies.

Senator FRIST. Mr. Chairman, can I make one other point?

Senator DURBIN. Sure.

Senator FRIST. Dr. Lumpkin, I love your analysis, the one in, is it 60,000?

Dr. LUMPKIN. Thirty-thousand.

Senator FRIST. Thirty-thousand mosquito bites. It puts it in an overall perspective. Could you help me understand, what is the bird doing? The bird is carrying the virus around. I was at the zoo, which is part of the Smithsonian Institution, at the end of July. While I was there, I had the opportunity to be with the head veterinarian while he was making rounds.

While we were there, someone brought in a bird. That was late July. That was before West Nile hit Washington, DC, and before the birds were found on the Capitol grounds. While we were making rounds to visit some of the other animals, someone brought in a second bird that morning, and then a third. Finally, it was clear that the birds were not from the same area, but there was something killing the birds. We did not know it was West Nile at the time. But with the test, it was proven to be West Nile.

There is a transmission cycle that incorporates both the mosquito and the bird. Does the titer, the level of the virus, have to get high enough that the bird dies? Could there be a number of birds flying around with West Nile, but only the ones with a high titer actually die?

Dr. LUMPKIN. I think it is even more complicated than that. It depends upon the bird species. Certain species—crows, blue jays—tend to be particularly sensitive to that. Other species will get infected, they will develop a massive viremia, viruses in the blood. Then they are bitten by multiple mosquitoes and that sort of potentiates the cycle.

What I do not think we fully understand is to what extent is the bird immune system part of the cycle that we see with St. Louis encephalitis and maybe other arboviruses, so that the experience in Illinois in 1975 was almost 600 cases in 1975, 19 cases in 1976. Could that have been also based upon some developing resistance amongst the bird population and will that have some impact upon West Nile? So I think we really need to understand better the biology in the bird, which clearly is a major player in this epidemic. It is primarily a disease of mosquitoes and birds and occasionally humans get in the way.

Senator FRIST. I have one more question.

Senator DURBIN. Sure. Of course.

Senator FRIST. This is switching gears. Currently, we are giving horse vaccine to birds today. Is there any science that the euine vaccine works for birds?

Dr. LUMPKIN. My understanding is that a number of zoos, including the Lincoln Park Zoo in Chicago, are experimenting with the bird vaccine. I do not know that they have published or they have had results yet.

Senator FRIST. The issue that many of you talked to is this whole idea of abatement. What is the appropriate Federal role in West Nile Virus, is it in vaccine development, as we talked about on the first panel? Does it relate to developing these diagnostic tests—either through mandates, or incentives to the private sector? Whatever it is, we have got to speed this system up as we go forward.

Similarly, on this panel, the issue of abatement is a critically important issue. That is on the front line. You are right there where it really matters, up front, and we are going to have to address it very soon. You are addressing the current crisis, but we also must have a strategy for next year. As we just heard, we do not know if this thing is going to get a lot worse or a lot better.

Dr. Gerberding outlined the Federal role, and she stressed the Federal role in planning, in counseling, in coordination of activities. However, the local responsibility focuses on the abatement because you are on the front line. You are the people who are out there who can best plan for a local community and who know what the needs are.

Then, there is the whole issue of resources. Is there a Federal responsibility for additional funding, given the increased funding through bioterrorism. As we all know, or as has been said repeatedly, surveillance, detection, response, communication, coordination is really hand-in-hand for both bioterrorism and West Nile Virus. With that increased funding, is it going to be redirected in some way for "dual-use" purposes related to West Nile?

That is going to be the debate that we are going to have. I tend to come out that mosquito abatement is a local issue in terms of support. But it is important that we use our Federal responsibility to support that local abatement on the issues of research, counseling, and coordination.

Just out of the interest of time, we do not need to go through that issue, but it is one that I think we are going to have to struggle with as we go forward.

Senator DURBIN. Thank you, Senator Frist. Senator Fitzgerald.

Senator FITZGERALD. Thank you, Senator Durbin.

Dr. Lumpkin, thank you very much for being here. You have really been on the front lines this summer dealing with the terrible situation we have in Illinois. I was struck that in your testimony you noted that about one-half of the cases in Cook County are concentrated roughly in the Oak Lawn and Skokie areas. You said that was the same areas that were most affected by the early 1970's outbreak of St. Louis encephalitis.

Is there any tracking being done of the ethnic origin of people who have had symptoms of the disease and then died from the disease? Is there perhaps a common genetic link? Do you think there is a missing gene in people who have died from this illness?

Dr. LUMPKIN. I do not think that we are in a position to answer that question. Some days, we have had so many cases, we have barely been able to determine the age and the county of origin of those cases. I think that is something we will have to look at over the winter.

Senator FITZGERALD. Are they tracking information about everyone who succumbs to this illness?

Dr. LUMPKIN. We are collecting information. I am not sure to what extent we are collecting ethnicity. Certainly, race is collected as part of our normal surveillance process.

Senator FITZGERALD. Is there something unique about the geography in those areas? I know Skokie is near the Skokie lagoons, although that is a little bit more to the east and north, I think, of the Village of Skokie. Those lagoons have a lot of water. It would seem to me that would be very good breeding grounds for mosquitoes. But on the other hand, I am struck that most of the cases are occurring in Cook County, which is unquestionably the most paved-over section of our State. I would think there would be a lot more mosquitoes in rural areas than there are in Cook County, Illinois. You have not drawn any conclusions, I gather, regarding where the disease is occurring in relation to the topography or geography of the area.

Dr. LUMPKIN. Obviously, that is something we need to study. When you look at the State, though, half of the people in the State live in Cook County and the close-in Chicago area, so it is not surprising. Again, when you look at the odds of one out of every 30,000 mosquito bites lead to a severe case of West Nile Virus, so if that is the case, more people are going to be exposed to mosquitoes. And while we think about Cook County being urban, one of the nice things about Chicago is that there is a lot of open space and there is a lot of park space, and so there is a lot of opportunity for mosquitoes to grow.

Unfortunately, though, the biggest problem, I think, with mosquito control is trying to get the message out. We had an entomologist up from the Centers for Disease Control the end of August to begin to address some of these issues and the first two homes that they went into, in the backyard, they found live mosquito larvae in containers in the backyards. And so there really needs to be a partnership between government and people to remove the breeding grounds, to take individual precautions, to make sure the screens are intact. This cannot be done alone by government. It really has to be a partnership.

Senator FITZGERALD. We had very heavy rains this past spring in Illinois, but then a fairly dry summer. That could play a role, too, could it not?

Dr. LUMPKIN. Certainly. In fact, the weather pattern that we had this summer was very similar to the weather pattern we had in 1975 and similar to the weather pattern they had in 1999 in New York.

Senator FITZGERALD. Illinois, at the end of the day, is somewhat similar to Louisiana, the other most affected State, in that we have a lot of standing water, and a lot of wetlands. They have bayous down there, and we had more wetland before Illinois was developed. But, we still have a lot today. I would think that the quantity of standing water that we have would make Illinois particularly vulnerable to infections that are borne by mosquitoes and make it likely that we would have mosquito control problems.

Dr. LUMPKIN. I think it is a combination of factors, and one of the issues that Senator Frist raised was about the Federal-State role. Clearly, we need assistance in doing that kind of research. We do not have the resources. We certainly do not have the scientific capabilities of NIH and so forth. So I think that is one of the things that we would really be looking for assistance, in trying to answer those questions, whether it be through satellite photos and analysis of the communities that are most involved versus another community, a case control study that way, as well as looking at issues related to the age of housing, whether or not gutters are collecting water in older communities. But why these communities and not the West side, the Western suburbs? I think we ought to try to figure that out.

Senator FITZGERALD. Dr. Houff, I was struck by your testimony that stated we are seeing different symptoms now, when the virus is present in a human, than we were a couple of years ago. You stated that you are seeing more neurologic symptoms. You described Parkinson's disease-like symptoms. It has been reported that there are polio-like cases of paralysis developing.

Do you think that when West Nile Virus first occurred on the East Coast a couple of years ago, we just were not looking for the virus as hard as we are today? Thus, could there have been cases with the neurologic symptoms you are describing now, but that they were not attributed to West Nile Virus? Or, do you think the virus is actually changing and it now is a little bit different than it was a couple of years ago?

Dr. HOUFF. With the caveat that what I said this morning is going to depend on collection of all the cases at the end of this and going back and looking, because obviously, this is the prospect I am looking at, I think that the clinical picture has changed and I do not think it is overlooking disorders in the New York epidemic. Probably we did, but let me give you an example of the negative.

In New York, clearly, paralysis and muscle pain was a prominent feature. In fact, in April of this year, when I gave a talk to the Chicago Medical Society, I told them I thought they might see this disease and I emphasized, look for patients with severe muscle pain and weakness. We have not seen that as much as we had in the past. So clearly, I think that it would be substantiated once we collect all the cases, that the neurological profile of what we see is changing.

Senator FITZGERALD. When you see paralysis in a patient who has West Nile, does that mean that the virus is settling in a nerve?

Dr. HOUFF. Well, if you look at the pathology, this virus is very prone to infect neurons, the neural cells that make the fibers that supply the muscles and the rest of the nervous system. It affects those cells more so than the supporting cells, like astrocytes and denticytes, the supporting cells of the brain. And so, yes, that is what you are seeing. You are seeing a cell that has been infected by the virus, a neural cell, and it is being destroyed by the virus. So that is why you see the absences.

Senator FITZGERALD. Have antiviral medications been tried on West Nile at all?

Dr. HOUFF. Ribavarin has been tried and showed promise in the test tube, but clinically, from all my knowledge, it has not been efficacious.

Senator FITZGERALD. Has it been tried in humans?

Dr. HOUFF. Yes, it has.

Senator FITZGERALD. It has? And it is just not effective?

Dr. HOUFF. It has been a disappointment, to say the least. The Israelis feel that, at least in some patients, they got worse using Ribavarin. But those studies are ongoing, and clearly, we do not have a treatment as yet.

Senator FITZGERALD. I see that my time is up. Senator Durbin, thank you.

Senator DURBIN. Thank you very much, Senator Fitzgerald. I might say that your comparison of Louisiana to Illinois was a much more pleasant idea before last Sunday's Bears game. [Laughter.]

Let me ask you this, and forgive me again, this person whose only academic exposure was biology for poets. If this question does not make any sense at all, please be kind. But is there any way of taking a fingerprint or DNA of this virus to try to trace it back in terms of its origin by country or other region, or is this—are we dealing with one single type of virus here that seems to be the culprit?

Dr. HOUFF. If you look at the genetic profile of this virus, it is almost identical to the isolate from Israel in 1988 and 1999, that was also present in geese, and I think that is interesting because geese there, avian species here, and different from the Romanian circulating virus. So clearly, you can do that. You can look at the genetic profile. All of the viruses that have caused human disease have been segregated in one lineage, lineage one. Lineage two is another genetic group of these viruses that have not been associated with human disease. And the isolates circulating in the United States, as far as I am aware, is, for all practical purposes, identical to the Israeli isolate in 1988 and 1999.

Senator DURBIN. Why do some mosquitoes carry it and others do not?

Dr. HOUFF. I think that is a critical question. If you—we do not know the answer to it, Senator. That is the first part of the question. But when we were talking about urban versus rural circulation of this virus, it is clear for West Nile and St. Louis, too, that there is a circulation in rural areas that is different in a species of mosquito and birds than it is in urban populations, and that appears to be the case for West Nile, also, certainly in Europe and probably in the United States. So I think those are areas that critically need study.

We just do not understand. To show you how little we understand—Dr. Fauci and I were talking about this—we do not know the receptors, for instance, where the virus gets into neural cells. We do not understand that yet. I mean, that is how basic we are.

Senator DURBIN. Let me just ask you to prognosticate, as Dr. Boozman has. I do not want to put words in your mouth, but you seem to feel that as far as Arkansas is concerned, you think next summer may be more challenging, not less. Dr. Fauci, I think, gave a guarded response saying he thought that—in fairness to him, I do not want to overstate it, but he thought that we may see a downturn in infection and death. Dr. Lumpkin, Dr. Houff, and Mr. Monica, if you would like to offer your opinion, too, I would appreciate your thoughts on it. What do you think that we face next year?

Dr. LUMPKIN. Again, it is going to be very difficult. New York, Florida, the following year after the large number of human cases had a reduction. In Illinois, with St. Louis encephalitis, we had a dramatic drop-off. We do not really know what our experience will be next year. I think we have to plan as if it is going to be as severe as this year and that is what our response is going to have to be based upon.

Senator DURBIN. Dr. Houff.

Dr. HOUFF. I would agree with Dr. Lumpkin. I think one thing we have not talked about, as this virus moves West and South, you are going to have naive populations that have never seen the virus before, and so I do not know whether you can compare Illinois to the West Coast, for instance. If you compare Illinois to New York, clearly, that is what happened. New York had a hit, then it reduced. Illinois started seeing birds last year and then we were majorly hit. I suspect that it may happen, as the virus moves West, we will see the same thing that has happened to Illinois in other areas of the country.

Senator DURBIN. Mr. Monica, do you have an opinion?

Mr. MONICA. Thank you. The trend the last 2 years has been an increase, so we have got to be on guard for that. It is important that we take all precautions that we can to educate our people and to put the controls in place to minimize that mosquito population. We just ask the Federal Government for support with funding for programs that local taxes, the ones that do not have a program can get one going and the ones that do have one, just support us in our effort to fight it.

Senator DURBIN. Thank you. My last question to Dr. Houff is, I am really intrigued by your observation concerning the Rockefeller Foundation's surveillance labs in other parts of the world and how that may be good harbingers of perhaps health challenges and public health trends. In your testimony, you have suggested that that program has been basically closed down and I wanted to ask, has any other entity stepped in in terms of academia or governmental surveillance labs in other parts of the world to share this information once the Rockefeller effort dissipated?

Dr. HOUFF. Senator, I am not aware of anyone stepping in to that degree. I think World Health has stepped in to some degree, and I discussed this before I came today with some of my colleagues with more experience with it. We all clearly believe that the dismantling of that warning system was detrimental to us.

Senator DURBIN. How long ago did that happen?

Dr. HOUFF. I believe it happened in the 1980's, the early 1990's.

Senator DURBIN. Thank you very much.

Did you have another question, Senator?

Senator FITZGERALD. Dr. Lumpkin, I want to go back to St. Louis encephalitis. Encephalitis is an inflammation of the brain. Does this condition occur after the infectious agent crosses the blood-brain barrier? Is that correct?

Dr. LUMPKIN. That is correct.

Senator FITZGERALD. Is the infectious agent in the case of St. Louis encephalitis a bacterium or a virus?

Dr. LUMPKIN. It was a virus that was essentially a kissing cousin of the St. Louis encephalitis virus.

Senator FITZGERALD. OK. So this is a very analogous——

Dr. LUMPKIN. I am sorry, of the West Nile——

Senator FITZGERALD. It is a flavivirus, correct?

Dr. LUMPKIN. Right, kissing cousins.

Senator FITZGERALD. OK. So this is a very similar disease. Did you say the St. Louis encephalitis started in Illinois in 1972?

Dr. LUMPKIN. No. In 1975, there was a major national outbreak, but most of the cases and the deaths occurred in Illinois. But it was a national outbreak.

Senator FITZGERALD. OK, and did it only last 1 year?

Dr. LUMPKIN. No. We have had periodic—because we do testing, we periodically find positive birds for St. Louis encephalitis and we have sporadic cases of St. Louis encephalitis in the State, a few cases a year, then we will have no cases, and then we will have three or four or five cases.

Senator FITZGERALD. So really, we only had a major problem in 1 year in Illinois, in 1975?

Dr. LUMPKIN. That was the big year, yes.

Senator FITZGERALD. And how many people contracted it?

Dr. LUMPKIN. Pretty close to—there were 590-some-odd cases and 47 deaths.

Senator FITZGERALD. OK. And so as of now, West Nile Virus is close——

Dr. LUMPKIN. It is very close. We are 518 cases and I was just informed we have now had a total of 29 deaths in Illinois.

Senator FITZGERALD. Did we spray heavily for mosquitoes at that time? I imagine we did. My impression is our mosquito abatement districts at the local level were much stronger in those days and had more resources.

Dr. LUMPKIN. They were. In fact, some of the news reports commented on the fact that when they were doing spraying from trucks in the Chicago neighborhoods this summer, that was the first time they had done that since 1975.

Senator FITZGERALD. OK. We have not had any discussion of the health effects of all these sprays, have we? We talked about that, I guess, while I stepped out.

The maps that have been given to us show that the livestock are heavily affected already out West, and while they show a large concentration of human cases in Illinois and the Midwest, the maps that were given to us do not show a great effect on our livestock. Would anybody care to comment, Dr. Houff or Dr. Lumpkin, about what we know about what has happened to cattle and hog populations?

Dr. LUMPKIN. The cattle and the hog population do not seem to be dramatically affected. The horse population in Illinois has been. We literally have hundreds of cases. The case fatality rate in horses exceeds 50 percent.

Senator FITZGERALD. The horses have to be vaccinated for some forms of encephalitis, do they not?

Dr. LUMPKIN. There is a vaccine for West Nile. It is available. It is a voluntary vaccine.

Senator FITZGERALD. Just for horses?

Dr. LUMPKIN. Just for horses. There is a multiple-dose course that is associated with that and you really have to be well into the course to be protected from—the horse has to be well into the course to be protected from West Nile.

Senator FITZGERALD. Now, with respect to our geese population in Illinois, my understanding is that they have not been dying from this virus, though many other birds have. But Dr. Houff, you said that this virus is very similar to a different virus that previously ravaged geese populations.

Dr. HOUFF. In Israel.

Senator FITZGERALD. In Israel.

Dr. HOUFF. Israel, correct.

Senator FITZGERALD. I wonder why it is not affecting the geese population now. It must be that there is some difference.

Dr. HOUFF. Whether those are analogous geese or whether they are genetically different, I do not know the answer. The virulence factors of the virus are poorly understood, and so we do not know why species are susceptible or immune or resistant to it. Clearly, if you look at the animal population in the United States who has never seen the virus, some of them are resistant. So either they have a brisk immune response or they cannot support the virus and its growth, and so we do not know that. And you can tell that even from animals that are susceptible.

In the crows, for instance, the virus rarely causes disease as much in the brain, and you look in the zoo population, the exotic birds, they get a massive encephalitis. So even in the bird population, the disease is different and we do not understand why.

Dr. LUMPKIN. In fact, in Illinois, we have not seen much amongst the Canadian geese, but the Lincoln Park Zoo had two red-breasted geese that did die from West Nile. So, again, it is going to be very closely associated with different species and sub-species of the avian population.

Senator FITZGERALD. Thank you all very much for your testimony. Thank you for being here, and good luck in your continued work on West Nile Virus.

Senator DURBIN. Thank you, Senator Fitzgerald.

If there are no further questions, this concludes the hearing. There may be additional questions submitted for the record for both panels.

In closing, I want to thank you and tell you how much we appreciate your sacrifice in coming here today. I think, based on the hearing that we have had, I am convinced that we need accelerated research in an effort to develop a test capable of large-scale screening in the U.S. blood supply for West Nile Virus and I think the FDA has testified and made it clear that we need to create some incentive for the private sector to meet this challenge.

We also need to provide the resources to share the testing with blood centers across America, so that once it is in place, that they can use it and can afford to do so. I believe we should be helping

States and localities, as we have this year with $29 million, and continue that effort so long as we are threatened by this and other mosquito-borne illnesses.

And finally, I think we need to try to accelerate, if we can, and it is a big "if," jump start the effort toward a human vaccine. The thought of waiting 3 years is troubling. Maybe that is the best that we can do. We certainly do not want to cut corners when it comes to public health and safety. But if there is a way for us to focus on this, I hope that we will.

Thank you to all our panelists for providing us insight today, and with that, the hearing is adjourned.

[Whereupon, at 12:22 p.m., the Committees were adjourned.]

APPENDIX

PREPARED STATEMENT OF SENATOR CLINTON

Thank you Mr. Chairman for taking this opportunity to examine this important issue. As you know, New York was the first state to be affected by the West Nile Virus in 1999. Since then we have been able to implement an effective system of disease surveillance, public education, and transmission control that serves as a model for other states that are only now having to deal with this new threat. Over the subsequent years, as a result of those efforts, we were able to reduce the number of infected persons and the number of deaths even as the virus spread to larger and larger areas of our state. Our experience shows that public health measures, when implemented correctly and adequately, can significantly reduce the harm this new disease can cause.

That said, this year, New York has seen a rise in the number of infections reported. Furthermore, we are now facing questions over the safety of our blood supply and life-saving organ transplants. These worrisome developments remind us of the critical need to support our current efforts and to redouble our search for even more effective remedies.

I am glad that you are all able to join us today and to provide us with a glimpse into the current and future work being done to protect our country from this new scourge. As much as we would like to wish it away, the West Nile Virus is here to stay, and it will take all of us working together to keep it from continuing on its destructive path.

PREPARED STATEMENT OF JULIE LOUISE GERBERDING, M.D.

Good morning, Mr. Chairmen and Members of the Committees. I am Dr. Julie Louise Gerberding, Director, Centers for Disease Control and Prevention. During my tenure as CDC Director, I am committed to achieving our vision of healthy people in a healthy world through prevention by a commitment to excellence in science, services, systems, and strategies. Thank you for your continued support and recognition of the critical need for a strong, flexible, well resourced public health system to deal with emerging threats, including bioterrorism and naturally occurring diseases such as West Nile Virus (WNV). I am pleased to be here to update you on CDC's public health response to WNV-related illnesses in the United States. I will also discuss the status of our WNV prevention programs.

Mosquito-borne illnesses in the United States were largely eliminated as a health risk in the middle of the last century, although mosquitoes that can transmit malaria, dengue, and yellow fever remain. Although Americans have not regarded mosquito-borne diseases as a major domestic threat for some time, the introduction and rapid spread of WNV has changed this. CDC has played an important leadership role in rebuilding the nation's capacity to monitor and diagnose mosquito-borne viral diseases through state and local public health partners around the country, but this year's events show that more work remains to be done. The more we strengthen our nation's front-line workers, whether in the field or in the laboratory, the better prepared we are to respond to new and emerging infections, such as WNV.

EMERGING INFECTIOUS DISEASE THREATS

The past decade has seen a significant number of emerging infectious disease problems in the United States. Some, such as E. coli O157:H7 and Cyclospora, are foodborne. Others, like hantavirus pulmonary syndrome, are transmitted from animals to people. Still others, like Lyme disease and ehrlichiosis, are vector-borne, while others, like vancomycin-resistant enterococci, result from the development of antimicrobial resistance in response to the misuse of antibiotics. Some emerging infectious diseases appear to be caused by new pathogens; others, in retrospect, have been here all along but were just not recognized. Some are clearly domestic in origin and others just as clearly have been introduced from abroad, illustrating the futility of thinking of infectious diseases in purely domestic or international terms. Infectious diseases know no borders. We must learn from the experiences of other countries in dealing with diseases such as bovine spongiform encephalopathy (BSE), variant Creutzfeldt-Jakob disease (vCJD), and foot and mouth epidemics in Europe, Ebola hemorrhagic fever in Africa, and avian influenza in Hong Kong.

CDC launched a major effort in 1994 to rebuild the component of the U.S. public health infrastructure that protects U.S. citizens against infectious diseases. In 1998, CDC issued Preventing Emerging Infectious Diseases: A Strategy for the 21st Century, which describes CDC's plan for combating today's emerging diseases and preventing those of tomorrow. It focuses on four goals, each of which has direct relevance to the detection of and response to WNV: 1) disease surveillance and outbreak response; 2) applied research to develop diagnostic tests, drugs, vaccines, and surveillance and prevention tools; 3) public health infrastructure and training; and 4) disease prevention and control. The plan emphasizes the need to be prepared for the unexpected whether it be the next naturally occurring influenza pandemic or the deliberate release of anthrax organisms by a terrorist. This CDC plan is available on CDC's website at www.cdc.gov/ncidod/emergplan/index.htm, and copies have been provided previously to the Committee.

Despite the diversity of emerging infectious diseases, public health workers, in partnership with health care providers in the United States, must detect them and respond. This is particularly true at the state and local levels of the system. CDC and other Department of Health and Human Services agencies have worked to strengthen the infectious disease public health infrastructure through cooperative agreements with states to build epidemiologic and laboratory capacity and through the development of emerging infections programs which are now in place in nine locations around the country. In many instances, these programs have significantly improved our ability to respond to infectious disease emergencies. Resources for bioterrorism preparedness and response have also bolstered capacity at the state and local level. But as highlighted by the Public Health Security and Bioterrorism Preparedness and Response Act, which originated in the Health, Education, Labor, and Pensions Committee and as illustrated by the challenges posed by the emergence of WNV, we still have gaps and needs to be addressed.

WEST NILE VIRUS

WNV is a mosquito-borne virus first recognized in the West Nile district of Uganda in 1937. Since then, it has been seen in Europe, the Middle East, Africa, and as far east as India. The virus lives in a natural cycle involving birds and mosquitoes, and only incidentally is transmitted to humans and other mammals, often in outbreak situations. A closely related virus, St. Louis encephalitis (SLE) virus, acts similarly in North America. Most humans who become infected with WNV through the bite of an infected mosquito will develop a mild illness or will not become sick at all. However, in a small fraction (<1%), encephalitis (inflammation of the brain) or meningitis (infection of the membranes surrounding the brain and spinal cord) will develop; approximately 10% of these patients will die. The elderly are recognized to be at higher risk than the rest of the population for the development of severe illness following WNV infection. It is likely that persons with compromised immune systems are also at higher risk.

The human and animal epidemic of WNV encephalitis which began in the northeastern United States in the summer and fall of 1999 underscored the ease with which emerging infectious pathogens can be introduced into new areas. The persistence of virus activity through 2002 indicates that WNV has become established in North America. This dramatic introduction and spread across the United States of a disease not previously seen in the Western Hemisphere reinforces the need to rebuild the public health system to prevent and respond to potential future introductions of other emerging infections.

WNV was recognized in the United States in late August 1999 when an alert infectious disease clinician at the Flushing Medical Center in Queens, New York, reported to the New York City Department of Health an unusual syndrome of fever and severe muscle weakness in several elderly patients. Eventually, 62 cases of human illness with WNV were recognized in the New York City area in 1999.

Laboratory studies of the virus demonstrated it was essentially identical to a WNV strain which had been isolated from geese in Israel in 1998, and all viruses identified in New York were indistinguishable by molecular typing techniques, indicating the outbreak resulted from a single introduction. When and how that introduction occurred is uncertain, but based on the wide circulation of the virus in the New York City area by August 1999, the virus likely was introduced several months earlier with subsequent unnoticed amplification in nature. Testing of a limited number of banked specimens from birds and humans have found no evidence of WNV in New York prior to 1999. Among the possibilities for how it was introduced are through an infected bird, through infected mosquitoes, or through an infected human.

In 2000, WNV was detected in 12 northeast and mid-Atlantic states. A total of 21 persons were found to be infected, 19 with severe illness and 2 with milder symptoms. Randomly conducted household surveys where residents were asked to provide blood specimens were conducted in Richmond County (Staten Island) and Suffolk County, New York, and in Fairfield County, Connecticut all areas with intense epizootic activity. Infection rates in the three locations were 0.46%, 0.11%, and 0%, respectively far lower than the 2.6% seen the year before in northern Queens. In 2001, 359 counties in 27 states and Washington, DC, reported WNV activity, including 66 human illnesses, to ArboNET, a web-based, surveillance data network maintained by 54 state and local public health agencies and CDC. This activity represented a marked increase from 2000 in both geographic range and number of cases.

CURRENT WEST NILE VIRUS SPREAD

This year, as you know, WNV infection has continued to expand geographically, reaching epidemic proportion in some states. As of September 22, 2002, surveillance in humans, birds, mosquitoes, and horses has detected WNV activity in 42 states and Washington, DC. Among humans, 1,672 cases with laboratory evidence of recent WNV infection have been reported from 31 states and Washington, DC. Among the 1,586 patients for whom data are available, the median age was 55 years, with age ranging from 1 month to 99 years; 855 patients were male; and the dates of illness onset ranged from June 10 to September 21. A total of 89 human deaths have been reported.

Building on lessons learned from the anthrax attack, we have activated our emergency operations center to coordinate our response, deploying field epidemiologists, vector-borne disease experts, and communications specialists to assist state and local health departments in the affected states in conducting surveillance, investigating cases, and implementing prevention and control efforts. As part of this effort, we have utilized the National Pharmaceutical Stockpile contract aircraft to rapidly transport specimens to CDC laboratories for diagnostic testing. In addition, we have provided education to health care workers, utilized the Health Alert Network (HAN) and the Epidemic Information Exchange(Epi-X) systems to disseminate information to clinicians and public health officials, and held press telebriefings all critical activities both for this disease outbreak and for strengthening our future response capabilities.

CDC, FDA, and HRSA, in collaboration with blood collection agencies and state and local health departments, are investigating a series of cases of WNV infections in recipients of organ transplantation and blood transfusion. An initial investigation in Georgia and Florida has demonstrated transmission of WNV in four recipients of solid organs from a single donor. The source of the organ donor's infection remains unknown and an investigation of the numerous transfusions of blood products that the organ donor received is ongoing.

Since the report of these cases, CDC has been informed of other patients with WNV infection diagnosed after receiving blood products within a month of illness onset. One of these patients also received an organ transplant. All of these patients resided in areas with high levels of WNV activity; investigations are underway to determine whether transfusion or transplantation was the source of WNV transmission. In each instance, precautionary measures, including withdrawal of unused blood products from donors whose blood was given to these patients, has been initiated.

WNV was isolated from a unit of frozen plasma that had been withdrawn as a result of one of these investigations. This finding indicates that the virus can survive in some blood components and probably can be transmitted by transfusion. In contrast, another investigation has found that a patient who received a unit of blood potentially-contaminated with WNV did not develop serologic evidence of subsequent WNV infection.

To better assess the risk of WNV transmission through blood transfusion or organ transplantation, CDC is actively engaged with FDA, HRSA, blood collection agencies, hospitals, and health departments to identify and follow-up additional possible cases. CDC has requested public health authorities to determine if persons reported with WNV infection donated or received blood transfusions or organs preceding their illness. Prompt reporting of these persons can facilitate withdrawal of potentially infected blood components. Additionally, the Public Health Service will work with industry to identify potential strategies to further increase the safety of the blood supply, including the development and application of assays that could be used to screen blood and plasma donations for WNV.

CDC studies have indicated that some patients with WNV infection have a syndrome similar to that caused by the polio virus. These patients can have paralysis of their arms or legs, and the paralysis can affect the muscles that control breathing. This finding is particularly important since many of these patients were being treated for Guillain-Barre syndrome—treatment which would have no benefit for a poliomyelitis-like syndrome and could lead to severe side effects. It is not known how long the paralysis will last; however, many patients did not significantly improve several weeks after disease onset. CDC is planning long-term follow-up studies of these patients.

PUBLIC HEALTH RESPONSE

After the outbreak of WNV in 1999, a West Nile Virus Interagency Working Group was formed to facilitate information sharing and coordination of activities among federal agencies with a role in monitoring and control. CDC leads the working group which includes representatives from the Departments of Agriculture, Commerce, Defense, and Interior, the Environmental Protection Agency, and the National Institutes of Health (NIH) who continue to monitor for WNV activity and seek ways to prevent future outbreaks, including research by NIH into the development of an effective vaccine and effective treatment. The working group routinely assembles for telephone conference calls and has provided several briefings to keep Congress informed of ongoing activities. CDC has also conducted weekly conference calls with our state partners to assure coordination of national surveillance.

As with many emerging infectious disease problems, addressing the WNV outbreak also requires a strong partnership between public health and veterinary agencies and the public. Effective systems need to be in place to ensure: 1) effective monitoring for WNV and other mosquito-borne diseases and 2) further development of prevention and control measures, including integrated pest management, public education, optimal mosquito control measures, vaccines and antiviral therapy. Further research on the basic biology of the virus and its natural ecology is also needed.

CDC has been the lead federal agency to respond to the WNV outbreak in humans. Since fiscal year 2000, DHHS and CDC have provided more than $58 million to state or local health departments to develop or enhance epidemiologic and laboratory capacity for WNV and other mosquito-borne diseases. In fiscal year 2002, approximately $35 million has been awarded to those public health agencies to address the continued spread of the virus.

CDC has also provided extramural funding to other federal agencies for related WNV surveillance and diagnostic activities in support of the states. A university-based research cooperative agreement was initiated in fiscal year 2001 to support studies on WNV distribution, pathogenesis, and variability and to provide training to future entomologists, biologists, and other vector-borne specialists. And, in fiscal year 2002, CDC will award funding to three educational institutions to initiate a program to train scientists in vector-borne infectious diseases. Finally, CDC has undertaken an aggressive intramural research program in several scientific areas to address the long-term needs related to epidemic WNV.

Surveillance, combined with professional and public health education, is the best strategy to confront the WNV problem. Among the recommended prevention measures to reduce the risk of exposure to WNV are 1) eliminating any areas of standing water around the house, i.e., draining standing pools, cleaning gutters, and emptying bird baths; 2) minimizing outdoor activities at dawn, dusk, and in the early evening; 3) wearing long-sleeved shirts and pants when outdoors; and 4) applying insect repellent according to package directions to exposed skin and clothing.

In addition to current activities, the following are some specific measures that CDC has implemented since the first WNV outbreak three years ago: developing the tests for use at state laboratories to diagnose WNV in humans, making and supplying the reagents used for these tests, and training every state laboratory in how to run them and how to diagnose infection; implementing Arbo-NET, an electronic surveillance system to track and monitor WNV and other mosquito-borne illnesses; convening a national meeting each year to provide public health workers, laboratorians, and local officials an opportunity to exchange the latest information about this disease; producing, in collaboration with partners, consensus guidelines for the surveillance, prevention, and control of WNV; developing educational materials for health care providers on the clinical aspects and diagnosis of WNV infection as well as public education materials; and assisting local officials with guidance on mosquito control.

CONCLUSIONS

In conclusion, addressing the threat of emerging infectious diseases such as WNV depends on a revitalized public health system and sustained and coordinated efforts of many individuals and organizations. As CDC carries out its plans to strengthen the nation's public health infrastructure, we will collaborate with state and local health departments, academic centers and other federal agencies, health care providers and health care networks, international organizations, and other partners. We have made substantial progress to date in enhancing the nation's capability to detect and respond to an infectious disease outbreak; however, the emergence of WNV in the United States has reminded us yet again that we must not become complacent. We must continue to strengthen the public health systems and improve linkages with health care providers and colleagues in veterinary medicine and public health. Priorities include strengthened public health laboratory capacity; increased surveillance and outbreak investigation capacity; education and training for clinical and public health professionals at the federal, state, and local levels; and communication of health information and prevention strategies to the public. A strong and flexible public health infrastructure is the best defense against any disease outbreak.

Thank you very much for your attention. I will be happy to answer any questions you may have.

PREPARED STATEMENT OF ANTHONY S. FAUCI, M.D.

Mr. Chairman and Members of the Committee, thank you for the opportunity to appear before you today to report on the state of West Nile Virus research at the National Institute of Allergy and Infectious Diseases (NIAID). Specifically, I will discuss our current research endeavors to address the diagnosis, prevention, and treatment of this disease, including our efforts to accelerate the development of a West Nile Virus vaccine. In addition, I will describe the Institute's future plans to accelerate and expand research on West Nile Virus within the context of the overall NIAID research program for emerging and re-emerging infectious diseases.

WHAT IS WEST NILE VIRUS?

I would like to provide a brief description of West Nile Virus, how it is transmitted, and its potential effects on the human body. The virus belongs to a group of disease-causing viruses known as flaviviruses, which are carried by ticks and mosquitoes. Other flaviviruses include yellow fever virus, Japanese encephalitis virus, dengue virus, and Saint Louis encephalitis virus. West Nile Virus represents an emerging infectious disease in the United States and has been isolated from more than 40 types of mosquitoes, primarily of the genus Culex, and from more than 110 species of birds.

West Nile Virus is transmitted to humans by infected mosquitoes, which generally acquire the virus while taking a blood meal from an infected bird. Although the entire spectrum of clinical disease in the United States has not been fully documented, data from outbreaks in the United States and elsewhere indicate that most infections in humans (80%) are asymptomatic. About 20% of infected individuals develop relatively mild symptoms that may include fever, headache, eye pain, nausea/vomiting and body aches, sometimes with skin rash and swollen lymph glands. If the virus crosses the blood-brain barrier, however, it can cause life-threatening encephalitis (inflammation of the brain) or meningitis (inflammation of the lining of the brain and spinal cord). The incubation period for West Nile Virus disease ranges from about three to 14 days.

NIAID WEST NILE VIRUS RESEARCH

Because of the outbreaks and subsequent deaths due to West Nile Virus infections since the virus was first detected in the United States in the summer of 1999, NIAID has reacted quickly to strengthen and enhance its West Nile Virus research portfolio. This effort is part of NIAID's comprehensive emerging infectious disease program, which supports research on bacterial, viral, and other types of disease-causing microbes.

Research is underway at NIAID to develop a vaccine, antiviral medicines, and new diagnostic assays for the West Nile Virus. Additionally, basic research is providing new clues about the virus itself, the disease in humans and animals, and how the virus is maintained in the environment. This knowledge is essential for the development of strategies to prevent, treat, and eventually control this disease. While we still have much to learn about the virus, the examples given below demonstrate the breadth and scope of NIAID's ongoing West Nile Virus research program and our commitment to maintaining and ultimately enhancing our role as a major player, in collaboration with the Centers for Disease Control and Prevention and the Food and Drug Administration, in combating this virus.

The major areas of NIAID's West Nile Virus research include: Basic research on the virus itself, on the disease in humans, and on its maintenance in nature—NIAID supports basic research to better understand the host, pathogen, and environmental factors that influence disease emergence. For example, basic research is helping scientists determine which flavivirus proteins contribute to the virus' ability to cause disease. Researchers also are investigating how protective immune responses are elicited within the central nervous system during acute flavivirus encephalitis. In addition, NIAID supports researchers who are investigating how West Nile Virus disseminates throughout the environment. The Institute's International Centers for Infectious Disease Research (ICIDR) program is supporting research in Mexico to study whether migrating bird populations carry the virus from its presumed point of entrance into the Western Hemisphere (New York City) to points in Central and South America. The emergence of West Nile Virus in these new areas, which harbor abundant mosquito populations, could provide conditions for a potentially severe epidemic.

Furthermore, researchers are examining the ecology and persistence of mosquito-borne encephalitis viruses, including the effect of genetic variation on the virus' spread and virulence and how birds might be year-round reservoirs for the viruses that cause encephalomyelitis. In addition, they are comparing the genetics of St. Louis encephalitis viruses from throughout California and different parts of the United States to determine the rate at which the virus is changing, and whether birds carry it between discrete geographic areas. The Institute also supports research to better understand the insects and ticks that transmit flaviviruses. Such an understanding will allow improved monitoring and surveillance, and enable the development and preliminary testing of strategies to control vectors of the virus.

Research to prevent and control spread of the disease—Since the first identified case in humans in the United States, NIAID has supported research to develop a candidate vaccine against West Nile Virus. This candidate vaccine is constructed using a licensed yellow fever vaccine as a backbone for the insertion of genes of the envelope of West Nile Virus and has undergone preclinical evaluations in hamsters, mice, monkeys, and horses. The company that developed the candidate vaccine, Acambis, is moving forward with Phase I trials, which are expected to begin in early 2003. NIAID intramural scientists have developed a West Nile Virus vaccine candidate, which they have tested in monkeys with promising results. This vaccine uses an experimental dengue virus vaccine as a backbone. Other approaches include a West Nile Virus DNA vaccine and one that uses expressed proteins. In addition, last year a hamster model of West Nile Virus was developed, which closely mimics human disease. The animal model will help accelerate the development and testing of new vaccines as well as antiviral therapies in humans.

Research to treat the disease—NIAID supports research to establish a system to screen chemical compounds for possible antiviral activity against West Nile Virus. Promising antiviral drug candidates will be tested in the hamster model. This resource allows scientists to evaluate a drug's safety and efficacy before moving on to possible human trials. Other research projects are investigating emerging diseases and developing candidate drugs to fight West Nile Virus. More than 300 drugs have been screened, and several have moved forward for preclinical evaluation. Research on immunotherapeutics (treatments that modify the body's immune response) also is being explored.

Research to improve detection and rapid diagnosis—Research is underway to allow for more rapid detection of West Nile Virus in samples from humans, including organs and tissues intended for transplantation, in other animals, or in vectoring mosquitoes. This research occurs mainly at small biotechnology companies attempting to develop new, commercially available diagnostic assays

Finally, the NIAID maintains the World Reference Center for Arboviruses at the University of Texas Medical Branch at Galveston. The Center has reference anti-West Nile Virus sera and seed lots of various strains of the virus. This international program involves characterizing viruses transmitted to people and domestic animals by mosquitoes and other arthropods and researching the epidemiology of arboviruses of the United States and overseas. During the last 3 years, these reagents have been provided on request to investigators in the United States and internationally.

RESEARCH OPPORTUNITIES FOR THE FUTURE

The NIAID has identified a number of opportunities for accelerating or expanding research to improve the diagnosis, treatment, and prevention of West Nile Virus. These areas include:

Basic Research:

The development of additional animal models, including primate models, for studies of viral pathogenesis and testing of new vaccines and therapies
Studies of correlates of immunity in the hamster model
Immune enhancement of pathogenicity (i.e. effect of prior immunity to other flaviviruses)
Characterization of severe and milder human disease and delineation of long-term central nervous system complications, including the effect of age on disease severity
Molecular evolution of the virus
Comparative virology between disease-causing flaviviruses

Diagnostics:

Development of diagnostic tools with improved specificity to eliminate cross-reaction with other flaviviruses
Development of a single diagnostic test that could be used for multi-species analysis

Prevention:

Evaluation of components of immune protection
Characterization of mechanisms of cross-protection between flaviviruses
Development and preclinical and clinical testing of candidate vaccines

Therapies:

Design and development of new antiviral medicines
Development and evaluation of immune-based therapies

Vector/Host/Ecology:

Molecular epidemiology (especially as virus "evolves" and spreads)
Basic epidemiology/natural history studies of the virus/host/vector and the establishment of important vector and host components of flavivirus cycling in North America
Development and testing of new and alternative mosquito control methods
Definition of viral epizootic/enzootic maintenance mechanisms
Development and assessment of modern methods to predict emergence and extent of spread of flaviviruses
Establishment/supplementation of overseas research programs in areas of intense flavivirus activity

FUTURE ACTIVITIES

New NIAID programs, such as the U.S.-based Collaborations in Emerging Viral and Prion Diseases and Partnerships for Development of Novel Therapeutic and Vector-Control Strategies, will increase research on West Nile Virus. Through partnerships with industry, the discovery and development of novel antiviral agents against West Nile Virus also will be expanded. Awards for these programs are expected in the early fall of 2002. In addition, many of the programs that have been recently developed and/or expanded to address biodefense in FY 2003, such as the In Vitro Antiviral Screening Program and the Cooperative Research for the Development of Vaccines, Adjuvants, Therapeutics, Immunotherapeutics, and Diagnostics for Biodefense, will support research on emerging infectious diseases such as West Nile Virus.

CONCLUSION

Mr. Chairman, despite our ongoing research efforts and early successes, we still have much learn about West Nile Virus. The NIAID will continue to expand its research portfolio to address all aspects of the virus to improve the diagnosis, prevention, and treatment of the disease. I hope that the information that I have provided here today has helped in the understanding of the virus and also has demonstrated NIAID's commitment to address this important public health issue.

————————

PREPARED STATEMENT OF JESSE GOODMAN, M.D.

Mr. Chairman and Members of the Committee, I am Dr. Jesse Goodman, an Infectious Diseases physician and scientist, and Deputy Director of the Center for Biologics Evaluation and Research (CBER) at the Food and Drug Administration (FDA or the Agency). I appreciate the opportunity to appear today to discuss FDA's response to the emerging threat of transmission of West Nile Virus (WNV) through blood and tissue. One of FDA's primary responsibilities is to help ensure the safety of the nation's blood supply. Within FDA, CBER is responsible for regulating blood and blood-related products. Our goal is to help ensure the safety of the nation's blood supply by minimizing the risk of infectious disease transmission and other hazards, while maintaining an adequate supply.

THE DEPARTMENT OF HEALTH AND HUMAN SERVICE'S (DHHS OR THE DEPARTMENT) COORDINATION

In 1995, DHHS created the Blood Safety Committee to ensure coordinated activities across the Department. Chaired by the Assistant Secretary for Health, the Committee includes the Commissioner of FDA, the Director of the Centers for Disease Control and Prevention (CDC), and the Director of the National Institutes of Health (NIH). There have been periodic meetings to discuss important safety and availability issues concerning the blood supply. On September 13, 2002, the issue of West Nile Virus was discussed with the Chair of the Blood Safety Committee. DHHS also established the Advisory Committee on Blood Safety and Availability (Advisory Committee) to look at broad issues including global public health, legal, ethical, and economic matters related to the blood system. On September 5, 2002, the issue of West Nile Virus was discussed at this Advisory Committee meeting so that the public and blood industry would be informed of the latest CDC and FDA efforts. In addition to these activities at the Department, the current status of the West Nile Virus epidemic was presented as an information item at FDA's Blood Products Advisory Committee (BPAC) on September 12, 2002. The BPAC considers scientific technical issues related to regulation of blood and tissue.

FDA'S ROLE

In recent years, tremendous steps have been taken that have greatly enhanced the safety of our blood supply. While we now face a new challenge, the American public can be assured that FDA is vigilant in its efforts to keep blood as safe as possible. In July 1997, CBER initiated a Blood Action Plan to increase the effectiveness of our scientific and regulatory actions and to ensure greater coordination with other parts of the Public Health Service (PHS). We recognized then, and recognize now, that potential threats to the blood supply will continue to emerge and we believe that helping to ensure blood safety requires timely action and a coordinated approach. Consequently, FDA works closely with CDC and NIH, and seeks input from consumers and the blood, diagnostic, and biomedical industries, to develop strategies that lead to appropriate studies, risk assessment, communication, and any other prevention strategies or regulatory controls needed to protect the blood supply.

Over a period of years, we progressively strengthened overlapping safeguards that protect patients from unsuitable blood and blood products. FDA's blood-safety system includes the following five measures; all of which are relevant as we address the threat of West Nile Virus.

Donor screening: Donors are provided educational materials and asked specific questions by trained personnel about their health and medical history. Potential donors whose blood may pose a health hazard are asked to exclude themselves. Donors also undergo medical screening to ensure that they are in good health at the time of donation.

Blood testing: After donation, each unit of donated blood undergoes a series of tests for blood-borne agents such as HIV-1, HIV-2, HBV (hepatitis B virus), HCV (hepatitis C virus), HTLV-1 and HTLV-II (Human T-Cell Lymphotropic Viruses), and the agent of syphilis.

Donor lists: Blood establishments must keep current a list of individuals who have been deferred as blood or plasma donors and check all potential donors against that list to prevent use of units from deferred donors.

Quarantine: Donated blood must be quarantined until it is thoroughly tested and the donation records have been verified.

Problems and deficiencies: Blood establishments must investigate any failures of these safeguards, and correct system deficiencies that are found by the firms or through FDA inspection. Firms must report to FDA any manufacturing problems, e.g. biological product deviations that may affect the safety, purity, or potency of their products.

If any one of these safeguards fails, affected blood products are considered unsuitable for transfusion and subject to recall.

WEST NILE VIRUS

Background

WNV is the most recent emerging infectious disease threat to public health and, potentially, to the safety of our blood supply. WNV primarily infects birds but can be transmitted to humans and other animals by mosquitoes. The majority of humans who become infected never develop symptoms. Approximately one in 150 of those people infected develop serious and life-threatening nervous system infection.

Although FDA was concerned about the possibility of West Nile Virus being transmitted by blood transfusions, until three weeks ago available evidence suggested that any risk was likely to be very low. We knew that such transmission was plausible because the virus is believed to be present in the blood for a period of a couple of days to weeks early in infection, including in patients who never develop symptoms of infection. Thus, a donor could feel well but, after mosquito exposure, could have the virus present in the blood for a short time and, while unaware of this, could donate blood. However, the risk of such an infected donor transmitting infection was believed to be very low because, unlike classic transfusion-transmitted viruses such as HIV and hepatitis B and C, where individuals may be infected for life, in West Nile infection there is no known chronic carrier state. Persons infected with WNV develop a rapid immune response, which clears the virus from the blood stream. Thus, to pose a risk to recipients, a donor would need to donate blood precisely during the days in which the virus is present in the blood.

In addition, levels of virus in the blood, when present, are low compared with HIV or hepatitis. Finally, despite three previous years of reported WNV cases in the United States, and many years of epidemic infections in other nations, no cases of transfusion transmission had been reported.

Risk to the Blood Supply

FDA has been working closely with CDC, state health departments, and blood organizations as part of the ongoing investigations of the recent WNV cases where patients had received organ transplants or blood transfusions. Based on the preliminary results of these investigations, we believe that it has been shown that organ transplantation can transmit WNV and that it is very likely that blood transfusion also has done so. Thus, there is a newly recognized threat to blood safety.

It is important to recognize that the true dimension of the risks of either blood transfusion or transplantation spreading West Nile Virus is not defined at this time and more information is critically needed. The risk could be higher or lower than the case reports suggest. Our investigations continue and new information, which shapes our understanding of the risk, comes to light almost daily. We are working closely with CDC, NIH, the Health Resources and Services Administration (HRSA), and with colleagues in the blood transfusion community to address this evolving situation, and to share new knowledge. We are communicating with Congress, the public, the media, the blood industry, and health professionals. As we have much to learn, we strive to present a clear picture of our evolving understanding of this potential risk.

To better define the risk and to determine what interventions are needed will require more knowledge. We are investigating case reports as they are received. We are also working with CDC, the blood community, and NIH to design and help implement studies that will give us a better idea of what proportion of donors may be infected in areas of differing intensity of disease transmission. We are hopeful that additional studies can provide information as to the degree to which such infection of donors then translates into risk for blood recipients. FDA also believes that studies are needed to confirm that long-lived blood stream infection (viremia) does not occur in persons who are potential blood donors. In addition, we are encouraging further studies of the effects on the virus on various conditions of blood product storage and manufacturing. We also are working with our partners to study the incidence of infection in frequently transfused individuals or those receiving plasma derivatives, such as patients with thallassemia, hemophilia, and immune deficiencies,

even though existing information indicates that steps normally taken in the manufacturing of plasma derivatives are expected to kill this virus, thus protecting recipients. All of this knowledge, as it becomes available, will help us, not only to better
understand the nature and the degree of any risk, but also to shape effective policy
and better protect the public.

While it is true that transfusion has not yet been conclusively proven to transmit
infection to any patients, we now believe, based on the aggregate of recent reports
and laboratory testing, that it is likely that this has occurred, and can occur in the
future. We are particularly concerned that in 1 of the cases under study, 3 different
donors, among 15 tested, may have carried the WNV at the time of donation. This
would obviously represent a far cry from the predicted likelihood of something like
1-2 in 10,000.

This estimate is from a CDC modeling study based on the density of infection during the 1999 epidemic in Queens, New York. Unanswered questions include: Is the
West Nile Virus persisting longer than expected in the bloodstream of some patients? Is there something unusual about the donors to this recipient? These possibilities are under investigation. Regardless of the answers, we now have a very
heightened level of suspicion and concern about all such reports, even if some may
represent coincidental occurrence of transfusion and infection. Such coincidences can
be expected to occur because the same individuals who need transfusions—the elderly, the chronically ill, and the immunosuppressed—are also most likely at higher
risk to develop severe West Nile infection.

FDA Response

Based on the growing distribution and increased number of cases of WNV in this
year's epidemic, FDA, working with CDC and NIH, decided it would be prudent to
issue an alert on August 17, 2002, to the blood banking community about the possibility of transfusion-transmitted WNV, and to emphasize the need for careful attention to screening procedures for blood donors, especially the exclusion of donors with
even mild symptoms that could represent early or mild WNV infection. In addition,
where there have been reports suggesting that recipients of blood transfusions may
have been infected by donated blood, we have worked with the blood banks and
state health departments involved to take a precautionary approach. In these cases,
the blood banks, at FDA's request, have withdrawn any untransfused blood components to protect other potential recipients while we investigate whether the donor(s)
may actually have been infected.

More recently, we learned that the Mississippi blood donor, who likely transmitted WNV to a transfusion patient, became ill four days after donating blood.
FDA policies encourage reporting by patients and resultant evaluation by blood
banks of such so-called "post-donation" events. We have alerted blood banks to this
finding and plan to issue guidance shortly to emphasize the importance of soliciting
and investigating post-donation reports of illness. In cases of serious illness, quarantine of blood products and investigation of the donor illness should provide an additional safeguard to reduce the risk to possible blood recipients. With regard to donors who never develop symptoms, we need to continue to investigate and collect
information so that we can develop appropriate policies to further reduce the risk
of transfusion-transmitted infection.

Some have raised the question whether not allowing anyone who reports mosquito
bites to donate blood would be appropriate. This would likely be both inefficient and
ineffective. Most people living in areas where WNV is spread will have had recent
mosquito bites and we would exclude a large number of safe donors for every one
donor with actual WNV infection. In addition, some individuals with WNV infection
will not recall mosquito contact. These factors suggest that such measures could create serious blood shortages with the potential to hurt far more people than might
be helped.

If areas of intense WNV transmission can be identified, another measure that
could be considered is excluding donors from those areas. This approach could potentially reduce risk, but the ever-expanding map of transmission makes it likely
that this approach could likewise cause blood shortages, yet may still fail to exclude
a significant number of infected donors. Nonetheless, if an unexpectedly high risk
is identified in a specific area, such measures could be considered, particularly if no
other effective interventions might be immediately available. It is also possible that
a greater use of autologous blood collections could be encouraged in areas of intense
infection.

The most effective means of reducing the risk of WNV transmission by blood
transfusion, if confirmed to be significant, would be to test donor blood samples for
the presence of the virus. Such testing could be performed generally (e.g., on all
blood donors nationally), which is most likely, or, if transmission is more restricted,

during seasons where transmission is occurring, or, in donors from selected regions. If specific populations (e.g., transplant or other immuno suppressed individuals) were to be identified as being at special risk for severe disease from receiving WNV infected blood products (and other populations not), donor screening could be performed to target blood intended for such individuals. It is unlikely, however, that an approach focused on specific recipients would be either desirable or practical, except perhaps as an interim measure were one needed until testing methods for broader use were made available. All individuals exposed to WNV are at risk for infection, and the elderly, who appear most at risk for severe disease, also need transfusions more frequently than other populations.

What are the prospects for availability of a good blood screening test for this disease? In short, the prospects are encouraging although it cannot happen overnight and significant challenges will need to be addressed. Classic tests for infectious agents involve looking for the human's immune response to the agent, in the form of antibodies. However, in the case of this virus, the WNV is present in the blood during the time period before antibodies develop. Therefore, direct methods to detect the virus itself will be needed. These methods are more complex, more expensive, and more difficult to implement on a broad scale than antibody tests. On the positive side, state and academic labs, some diagnostic companies, and the CDC, have developed sensitive tests that can amplify and detect the genetic material of this virus.

Tests based on similar technologies, called NAT (for nucleic acid amplification test), are now universally used in the U.S. to test all donated blood for the presence of early HIV and hepatitis C infection. These tests have helped make our blood supply very safe from these infections, with risks of transmission of these agents in the 1/1,000,000 range for hepatitis C and in the 1/2,000,000 range for HIV. The medical diagnostics industry, the blood industry, and FDA have significant expertise in the development, implementation, and evaluation of NAT testing. Such experience will be useful in adapting WNV test methodologies currently in use in diagnostic laboratories to more widespread and automated use for blood screening. There are many challenges, including the need to achieve high levels of reliability when used in populations with very low frequencies of infection, the lower levels of virus compared to those currently tested, the difficulties involved in scale-up, and time needed for test development and wide implementation. For testing organ donors, special challenges would be added, including timing, logistics, and determination of whether screening blood samples can rule out infection in tissues and organs. While we do not yet know if screening of blood will be needed, we believe it is likely, and therefore most prudent, to move forward to facilitate its availability as soon as possible.

To this end, we are working with our partners in the blood and diagnostics industries, including the American Association of Blood Banks and AdvaMed. Recently, they hosted an important meeting with FDA, CDC, and state health departments with potential WNV diagnostics methodologies to discuss the development of assays of potential utility, to stimulate interest in testing, identify barriers and approaches to resolve them, and foster technology transfer and sample sharing, all in an effort to get all partners the information and materials needed to be as prepared as possible to meet the potential need for testing. This meeting was quite successful and we plan a follow-up public workshop at FDA co-sponsored by CDC, NIH, and HRSA in the near future. Further development and implementation of effective screening tests for WNV will depend in large part on the efforts and innovation of our public health and blood and diagnostic industry partners. It is important to note, however, that FDA can use its regulatory authority to make such tests available even before licensure under an investigational new drug (IND) application. Again, while we hope that this will not turn out to be needed, we must be prepared.

One final approach that could be used in helping to address the WNV threat, as well as other future and potential infectious risks to the blood supply, is called "pathogen inactivation." In pathogen inactivation, a chemical and/or physical treatment of blood products is used that is capable of killing many infectious agents. FDA recently held a workshop on this promising and innovative strategy. Several approaches are currently under study and may be effective at inactivating viruses such as WNV. Although promising, it is important to realize that preventive treatment of blood products affects the products given to all recipients. In other words, if only 1 in 5,000-blood units had an infectious agent present, for every patient protected from the disease, 4,999 would receive a product that may be altered in some ways that could affect its other characteristics and, perhaps, its safety. For these reasons, these approaches must be, and are being, carefully evaluated for their immediate and long-term safety. However, should WNV risk prove significant in degree, or blood screening be difficult to implement in a timely manner, pathogen inactivation may prove valuable as an approach to reducing risk in blood either from high risk areas and/or potentially for blood being given to recipients at highest risk of developing severe disease. Such approaches could also be initiated and evaluated in pre-licensure pilot studies under an IND application. FDA is also currently planning to specifically address the inactivation of WNV by such methods in conjunction with its upcoming workshop on WNV donor blood testing.

Treatments for WNV and Vaccine Development

Most people who become infected with WNV will have either no symptoms or only mild ones. More severe disease occurs in approximately 1/150 of those infected and is manifested as encephalitis, meningitis, or meningoencephalitis. Encephalitis refers to an inflammation of the brain; meningitis is an inflammation of the membrane around the brain and the spinal cord, and meningoencephalitis refers to the combination of both. There are currently no drugs on the market to treat this virus. There are currently six IND applications involving two products in effect at FDA for the treatment of WNV. The National Institute of Allergy and Infectious Diseases (NIAID) has also supported promising research to identify and develop potential treatments for this disease.

While there is currently no licensed vaccine available to prevent WNV infection, FDA is aware of several promising approaches to vaccine development and believes that this is a potentially viable strategy to address this increasing public health threat. Because of the increased presence of WNV in the U.S., NIAID has supported research in this area. NIAID announced that in 1999 it funded a fast-track project to develop a candidate WNV vaccine with Acambis PLC. Scientists at CBER are also engaged in studies, which may hold promise for developing a vaccine effective against WNV.

Given the important and increasing public health impact of WNV infection, including the potential threat to blood safety, and the lack of available vaccines and therapeutic measures, FDA places a high priority on facilitating the development and review of such products.

CONCLUSION

As we act on our current knowledge of the risk of WNV to the blood supply, and share information with the public as it becomes available, it is also important that we keep the risk, even a risk that is not yet well understood, in perspective. There has been a remarkable decrease in the transmission of viral diseases through blood in recent years. We believe that our experience in dramatically reducing the risk from HIV and hepatitis will serve us well in addressing whatever needs to be done with respect to the challenges we now face with the WNV. Thousands of individuals' lives are saved or transformed every year by organ transplants. Millions of lives are enhanced by transfusion of blood and related products. It is essential that we keep these medical procedures and related products as safe as possible.

We will continue to work closely with our partners in CDC, NIH, HRSA and the states, and to engage the blood and diagnostics industries to harness their capabilities to help make a sensitive blood test a reality. We will continue to share information with and seek input from the public and from experts outside of government, as we recently did with both FDA's Blood Products Advisory Committee and the DHHS Advisory Committee on Blood Safety and Availability. We will continue to engage the highest levels of attention with the Department, including discussion of major blood safety policy issues with the Assistant Secretary's Blood Safety Committee.

As a final note, FDA would like to encourage the public to continue donating blood because supplies are low and the need is great. Blood remains in short supply, in part, because of the extensive safety measures already in place. Some people are concerned that they might get an infection by donating blood. We want to assure you and the public that donating blood is a safe procedure. We also want to take this opportunity to thank blood donors and to emphasize that the cornerstone of our blood safety system is the volunteer blood donor. Thank you very much for the opportunity to testify today.

I welcome your ideas and your questions.

PREPARED STATEMENT OF SIDNEY ANDREW HOUFF, M.D.

The outbreak of West Nile Virus (WNV) infections in the United States has challenged government, medical and veterinary resources. The rapid geographic expansion and persistence of the virus in newly established enzootic areas in North America indicate WNV has become permanently established in the United States (1). Renewed efforts to understand human disease and the biology of the virus will be necessary as we are likely to continue to experience outbreaks of WNV for the foreseeable future.

I have divided my testimony into two areas. I will first address the clinical features of WNV infections in humans including our experience in 2002. I will then turn to the biology of WNV. Here I will describe additional studies of WNV that will be required to address the needs of populations at risk of infection, including domestic and wild animals.

The response of the Centers for Disease Control and Prevention and the Illinois Department of Health have been outstanding. Both federal and state agencies have provided needed information in a timely manner to physicians and other health care providers grappling with patients with WNV. Essential information has been presented on the Internet, allowing easy access to health care providers. In Illinois, we have been able to access up to date information on human and animal infections. CDCP and IDPH sites have offered valuable information for submission of specimens for testing and other essential information needed by health care providers. At Loyola University Medical Center various avenues of communication have been used to provide the latest information on WNV to attending and resident physicians, nurses, and allied health personnel. A "high index of suspicion" for WNV infection has been instituted to assure cases of infection are not overlooked. The Department of Neurology at Loyola University Medical Center has developed protocols to assure WNV infection is considered in the differential diagnosis of patients with neurological syndromes other than meningitis, encephalitis and meningoencephalitis.

Clinically, West Nile Virus infection usually results in an unapparent infection in humans (1). A serological survey for WNV antibodies conducted in New York City in 1999 found that approximately 20% of persons infected with WNV had developed West Nile fever. Most patients who developed symptoms often complain of the sudden onset of fever, malaise, anorexia or loss of appetite, nausea, vomiting, eye pain, headache, muscle pain, skin rash and lymphadenopathy (swollen lymph nodes). The risk of developing serious neurological disease is based on experience in previous WNV outbreaks in Romania, Israel and New York City. In the Romanian outbreak of 1996, 1 in 140 to 320 infections led to disease of the nervous system. In New York, 1 in 150 infections resulted in neurological disease. The experience in Israel is similar to that seen in New York City. These findings suggest that the WNV strain circulating in the United States and Israel is associated with a higher rate of neurological infections. Meningoencephalitis, encephalitis and meningitis have been the predominant forms of neurological disease associated with WNV infection (2). Profound muscle weakness and muscle pain have been a prominent feature in WNV outbreaks in the United States (3).

Our experience suggests that nervous system infection with WNV during 2002 may have several unusual features. The profound myalgias encountered in New York City in 1999 and subsequent outbreaks in 2000 and 2001 have not been a prominent feature of our cases in 2002. We have also encountered involvement of the optic nerve and basal ganglia more frequently than expected. Whether or not our experience reflects a true change in the clinical features of WNV meningoencephalitis must await more extensive study of the clinical features of cases seen in 2002. If the clinical features of WNV meningoencephalitis are indeed changing, it will be important to recognize these changes as we confront future outbreaks of WNV infection.

Treatment for West Nile Virus infection has been limited to supportive measures to control cerebral edema, seizures, and systemic complications of the infection. Ribavirin in high doses and Interferon-a are effective in vitro (4). Control studies have not yet been completed for either agent. One patient has been treated with intravenous gamma globulin containing high antibody titers to WNV (5). The efficacy of intravenous gamma globulin cannot be determined from this one case.

Hyper immune gamma globulin with high antibody titers to WNV could offer an additional treatment for WNV neurological infections. Antiviral antibody therapy has been shown to be effective in experimental and human virus infections of the central nervous system. Antibody treatment of mice with Sindbis virus infection of the brain results in clearing of virus from neural cells. Humans with hypogammaglobulinemia who develop central nervous system enterovirus infections have been successfully treated with hyper immune gamma globulin. Gamma globulin therapy can be instituted without the long delays required for drug development. Individuals infected with West Nile Virus during the 2002 outbreak are likely to have high titers of antiviral antibodies in the serum. These patients could serve as donors for hyper immune gamma globulin that can then be stored for use in future outbreaks of WNV infection. The genetic stability of WNV suggest antibodies generated during the 2002 outbreak should be effective in neutralizing WNV in outbreaks in the near future.

West Nile Virus presents a serious threat to human health for several reasons. Many, including some members of the news media, underestimated the magnitude of the problem at the beginning of the epidemic when only a small number of human cases had appeared. The current 424 human cases and 22 deaths in Illinois illustrate the difficulty in predicting the seriousness of these epidemics.

Experience over the last 4 years suggest that we are likely to see continued outbreaks of WNV infection. The spread of the virus across the United States will likely be followed by new outbreaks of WNV infection in humans and animals. Spread of the virus to Canada, Central and South America by migrating birds will place additional human populations at risk of disease. The WNV strain circulating in the United States appears to have a higher rate of neurological infections than those seen in Romania and other areas of the world. Viral evolution can result in changes in virulence, disease pattern, host cell range, and other properties of the virus. While it is true that viruses transmitted by insects to mammals are constrained in their ability to mutate, the possibility of changes in the virus are real and require study. Transmission of WNV by unusual means such as blood and organ transplantation are of uncertain significance at the present time. However, since most patients with WNV infection are asymptomatic, these individuals would not provide a history to blood collection agencies that would preclude their donation of blood and blood products. It is important, therefore, to determine the risk of transmission from patients with asymptomatic infection to better assess the risk to the blood supply.

Although much is known about arthropod transmitted virus infections in humans, we also have much to learn. The epidemiology, wildlife enzootic cycles, and the pathogenesis of animal and human disease of WNV are important areas requiring further study. The enzootic cycle of virus circulation is a critical factor in the biology of virus transmission. A rural or sylvatic cycle of wild birds and ornithophilic mosquitoes and an urban cycle with domestic birds and mosquitoes feeding on humans and birds support WNV transmission. Illinois offers an excellent site to study wildlife factors involved in outbreaks of arthropod transmitted neurological diseases. The state has experienced significant outbreaks of both Saint Louis Encephalitis virus and WNV infection. Elucidation of the factors that support these outbreaks in Illinois may provide valuable information that will be applicable in other regions of the country.

The molecular biology of WNV also needs further study (6). The strain of WNV circulating in the United States originated in Israel. It has several unique properties. For instance, high avian mortality has only been encountered in outbreaks of WNV in the United States and Israel. The rate of neurological disease also appears to be higher in urban outbreaks of WNV compared to those in rural areas. The viral properties responsible for these and other features of WNV infection are only beginning to be understood. Continued efforts are needed to define viral factors associated with virulence, host cell range, and the possibility of viral persistence. The evolution of WNV strains in nature may help us understand how viruses "jump" to other species and present new threats to human health. The immune response to WNV infection is also an important area of future study that will be important in attempts to control virus replication in infected patients.

A multidisplinary approach will be needed if we are to understand the challenges of outbreaks of arthropod transmitted infections such as WNV. The Conversation Medicine Center of Chicago is a collaborative effort of Loyola University Medical Center, the Brookfield Zoo, and the University of Illinois that includes physicians, veterinarians, entomologists, field biologists and others. The Center is currently examining areas of research that would benefit from the collaborative expertise of its members. The enzootic cycle for WNV is one important area of interest. Isolation of WNV from squirrels and dogs suggest the virus is spreading to other mammalian species during the 2002 outbreak. Infection of other mammalian species has been noted in past outbreaks. In most species WNV infection does not result in titers of WNV sufficient to serve as a source of infection for mosquitoes or ticks. However, lemurs in Madagascar and several reptile species have been shown to develop virus titers in the blood that are sufficient to infect mosquitoes. Surveys need to be conducted to determine which species have been infected during the 2002 outbreak and if any support virus replication to levels sufficient to infect mosquitoes. If such species are found, the range of mosquito species infected with WNV may increase. Additional studies of WNV infection in mosquitoes, evolution of WNV strains in the laboratory and nature, and the factors associated with spread of infection to incidental hosts are currently being discussed. We are currently finishing a submission to study the pathogenesis of WNV infection in the brain in experimental animals. We believe the multidisplinary approach used by the Conservation Medicine Center of Chicago and other such groups around the country offer the best opportunity to successfully address the challenges of WNV and other vector borne diseases.

The experience gained meeting the challenges of WNV outbreaks will improve our readiness to successfully address the challenges of bioterroism. Many of the same technological and epidemiological approaches used in the investigation of the WNV outbreak will be helpful in the event we are attacked using similar agents. I would also suggest consideration should be given to reopening surveillance laboratories, such as those supported by the Rockefeller Foundation. These laboratories closed during an era of increased international travel and increased risk of emerging infections, provided vital information for the study and control of insect borne viruses. Reestablishing surveillance laboratories that can warn the emergence of known viruses or new viruses will be invaluable in the future.

In closing, I wish to thank the committees for the opportunity to present my views. I look forward to answering any questions you may have at the hearing on September 24, 2002

PREPARED STATEMENT OF JOHN R. LUMPKIN, M.D.

First of all, let me thank the Committees for this opportunity to provide testimony on West Nile Virus and it's very real and devastating effect in Illinois. As one of the States hardest hit, Illinois has been working hard, using every available resource, to make an impact on stopping the spread of West Nile. I am hopeful that my testimony can shed some light on our activities and the needs of our State, and probably other states that are impacted by this disease.

I know that there are specific questions of interest to committee members but, I would like to begin with some background on our experience in Illinois. As you probably know, Illinois, Louisiana, Ohio, Michigan, and Mississippi have reported the most cases of WNV during 2002.

In Illinois cases have been reported in 38 of the 102 counties (approximately ⅓ of the State). Through 9-20-02 Illinois has reported 473 cases including 25 deaths (this is a moving target) Although we have no hard data, numerous survivors have not been discharged to their homes, but to long-term care facilities or rehab facilities. We understand a major (at least short term) sequella is inability to ambulate

The majority of cases have been in the Chicago metropolitan area. In the Chicago metropolitan area, two areas of suburban Cook County bordering the City of Chicago (Oak Lawn vicinity and Skokie vicinity) have been over-represented in the case count.

IDPH has actually planned for WNV since summer 2001. Included in the Department's FY02 budget was an initiative related to West Nile. IDPH provided funding to allow a number of local health departments to develop their own plans to ensure coordination of efforts with municipalities, mosquito abatement districts, street departments or other entities that would be involved in such an endeavor.

Infections in Illinois were unlikely prior to 2002. The virus was first documented to be present in Illinois in September 2001 when there was evidence in dead crows. Not much time remained in the mosquito feeding season after discovery of WNV in Illinois in 2001 but the evidence of it's presence started our preparations in earnest.

Realizing the potential impact, Governor George H. Ryan created a Cabinet level work group, headed by IDPH, to coordinate the state's response among the various agencies involved which included the Department of Agriculture, Natural Resources, Environmental Protection and Public Health.

The Work Group has been meeting consistently since the early Fall of 2001, and more recently, talking on a daily basis to coordinate our efforts and information.

In more general terms, a plan for surveillance of human mosquito borne infections was established in 1976 and has been implemented annually since that time.

CURRENT EFFORTS TO CONTROL THE SPREAD OF WEST NILE VIRUS IN ILLINOIS

After WNV was first detected in wild birds in Illinois in May 2002, IDPH put out press releases concerning personal protection and the removal of standing water and produced 30,000 color posters and fliers, over half of which have been distributed to local health departments and others that request them. Bulletins were issued to all local health departments and municipalities recommending that at minimum, larvicide be applied to street catch basins twice during the summer to prevent an outbreak of WNV.

Prior to the first human case of WNV, Public Health awarded $264,059 to 20 local health departments to prepare for the expected WNV outbreak in Illinois. The grants allowed many LHDs to train their personnel, provide information about WNV to municipalities, and make contacts with mosquito control agencies.

An additional 18 grants totaling $462,490 have been made to LHDs to create vector control programs and cleanup mosquito-producing tire sites.

Within a week of learning of the first Illinois resident to contract WNV on 8/8/2002, the Governor instituted daily meetings of the four-state agency WNV Task Force, created in 2001, to make funds available to local agencies to combat the advance of WNV in Illinois. Within 3 weeks, the first emergency grants were executed.

Since then, emergency WNV mosquito control grants have been offered to 37 local health departments where human WNV cases have occurred of which 24 departments have requested and received grants totaling about $2.6 million providing protection for about 8.1 million people.

Due to the shortage of licensed mosquito control personnel in Illinois, the Department of Agriculture, in cooperation with Public Health, issued an emergency rule to allow health department and municipal officials to apply certain mosquito larvicides, without a license, after attending a one-hour seminar. Public Health staff have offered over 20 emergency-rule larviciding seminars to over 500 local officials.

Public Health has provided extensive technical assistance and advice to local health departments on mosquito control and is working closely with CDC and DNR and the UI Vet School to determine the etiology of WNV, especially concerning the two clusters of cases that have occurred near Chicago, and possible reservoirs and hosts.

Public Health has responded to thousands of phone calls, e-mails and news media contacts to answer questions from the media and the general public.

What more can federal and state governments do to prepare for next summer?

However, we believe that Increased attention in the form of federal funds are needed at both the state and federal level for more full-time Public Health staff to:

Administer a grant program to assist local health departments in assuring that arbovirus surveillance and control programs are provided where these services are not offered by mosquito abatement districts or other agencies.

Work with mosquito abatement districts and other municipal mosquito control programs to assure the implementation of comprehensive and effective mosquito control programs next spring that emphasize source reduction and larviciding.

Provide mosquito control training for local health departments and municipalities that leads to licensing by the Department of Agriculture; and training in mosquito and bird collection techniques to assist Public Health in arbovirus surveillance work.

Provide resources to state public health, animal disease, and research laboratories to provide the analytical, entomological, and epidemiological tools needed to fight WNV, as well as funding for materials and personnel to rapidly perform confirmatory testing

Additional surveillance staff are also needed that can be mobilized to facilitate rapid processing of human surveillance data, rapid analysis of data and rapid dissemination of data.

Begin early public information campaigns.

We also believe that USEPA should consider the creation of a special Pesticide Applicator license for municipal officials. Current licensing focuses on agricultural pesticide applications. The license should only require enough training so that municipal officials could apply low-risk mosquito larvicides.

Have State resources to fight West Nile Virus come at the expense of other programs?

Local Health Protection Grants, intended to support local health department programs in water supply, sewage disposal, food sanitation and infectious diseases were used to support the emergency WNV mosquito control grants provided by the WNV Task Force to LHDs.

Public Health staff that operate other programs dealing with general administration, lead, mold and moisture, environmental toxicology, and structural pest control have been diverted to WNV response.

Federal money to support bioterrorism preparedness, epidemiology and laboratory capacity, has made us better prepared to deal with this outbreak. Specifically, we believe this has been demonstrated with enhanced rapid communication to LHDs, hospital ICPs, hospital laboratories and infectious disease physicians and the funding used in disseminating information about responsibility to report human infectious disease cases responsibilities and methods of reporting

Where have West Nile Virus infections been most prevalent in 2002, and why have infections become significantly more common this year, as compared to years past? Can we expect the number and severity of human cases to worsen in years to come?

The virus has expanded its range across the Midwest into areas that include large population centers, such as Chicago, suburban Cook County and the nearby suburban counties. Although the virus first appeared in Illinois during August 2001, it was near the end of the mosquito transmission season. Apparently, in 2001 virus amplification in wild birds did not reach a level where humans were at significant risk.

In contrast, WNV-positive dead birds appeared in May 2002, at the beginning of the summer, which permitted summer-long virus amplification in the wild bird population. Furthermore, the hot summer of 2002 was conductive to breeding and flight activity of the house mosquito, the primary vector of WNV. As a result, there was a high level of virus amplification in birds and mosquitoes. Consequently, more people were exposed to the virus in 2002.

Is West Nile Virus similar to any other mosquito-borne illnesses found in the United States? If so, what lessons has the Department learned from responding to previous outbreaks?

WNV has many similarities to St. Louis encephalitis, which caused an outbreak in Illinois during 1975. Since then, cases of SLE have been rare in Illinois, although they have been more common in southern states.

However, WNV appears to be better adapted to the temperatures in northern states; it has even been detected in southern Canada.

Because there have been few cases of mosquito-borne disease in recent years, many local mosquito abatement programs have been reduced or eliminated, which results in less effective emergency control programs. Similarly, there are few environmental staff with experience in mosquito surveillance and abatement at the state level to assist local officials during emergencies.

State and local mosquito abatement resources need to be rebuilt.

A lesson learned from the SLE outbreak of 1975 was to establish a system for surveillance of human illnesses before cases occur. In Illinois we have such a system in place.

Another lesson learned was to establish an "early warning system" that became functional in 1976 to detect evidence of arbovirus infections in wild birds. IDPH also has this type of system in place. The Department has traditionally collected some 5000 live birds annually for testing. The bird blood is tested for SLE, EEE and now, WNV. Additionally, we test mosquito pools as a supplement to live bird testing.

Provide scientifically sound information to organizations that provide mosquito control services on appropriate mosquito abatement practices.

Our ability to identify and track disease is key to being able to take appropriate measures. In addition to that very real part of the equation—both government and individuals can do a lot to curb the spread of the disease by specific activities. Comprehensive mosquito abatement programs are important to addressing the problem. But what remains the single most effective precautions are those that can and should be taken by individuals:

Stay indoors at times when mosquitoes are most active when outdoors—wear protective clothing.

Use mosquito repellent containing 25-35% DEET.

Check residential screens to ensure insects are kept out of living areas and, eliminate stagnant water where mosquitoes might breed.

PREPARED STATEMENT OF NICKIE MONICA

Thank you Mr. Chairman and Members of the Committee. I am Nickie Monica, Parish President of St. John the Baptist Parish, a residential suburb of the New Orleans Metropolitan Area. St. John Parish's population is nearing fifty thousand residents and it is one of the fastest growing areas of Louisiana. St. John Parish is located on the Mississippi River which has a substantial industrial job base that has brought significant economic development and higher than average wages for its residents.

It is indeed a pleasure to appear before your subcommittee to shed some light on a growing local problem that has national implications. Just a short time ago, mosquitoes, like any other insect, were just another nuisance that interrupted the outdoor life of residents who live a tropical climate. Unfortunately, it has now been thrust into the national media because it has become a serious health hazard with devastating consequences to many families around this country, including those in my state of Louisiana. Fortunately, Mr. Chairman, St. John Parish has not yet experienced a human fatality—something I believe is due to our proactive measures to combat this growing public menace. However, if a more prominent effort is not put forth, I am fearful that it is just a matter of time before tragedy strikes home.

St. John the Baptist Parish instituted its own regimented mosquito program over a decade ago as an added quality of life issue for its residents. The program is run by professional and licensed entomologists who are experienced in the field of serveilance and treatment. Our spraying and treatment program experienced no problems until the West Nile Virus began approaching Louisiana from the East Coast states. We immediately allocated 30 percent more funding to the spraying program without additional surveillance. We also began a public awareness campaign to encourage residents to minimize the threat of larvae hatchings around homes and businesses. Additionally, the Louisiana Department of Health and Hospitals instituted statewide Public Service Announcements reminding all residents to be vigilant and lessen the threat of infection. In my opinion, this has been effective in itself.

Even though St. John the Baptist Parish has an adequate control program in place, our financial ability to continue to fight over a sustained period of time is practically exhausted. We all know this problem is not going away. The question is how best to "fight and fund" an effective program. The fact that parishes and cities that do have programs also have West Nile Virus is of a great concern. Mr. Chairman, I know my own parish and state best and have thoughts on how to provide a remedy and abate danger. We now have to look to the experts to tell us what is the best protocol that can be implemented statewide. It is definitely more than a local problem. It is a national and state health concern, and the federal government does need to play a major role in "fighting and funding." Of course, any federal program must be consistent statewide in order to maximize effective abatement efforts.

Mr. Chairman, I also, want to thank the Louisiana Congressional Delegation and the United States Congress for their efforts to assist Louisiana and the rest of the affected areas of the country in this effort. For example, further federal assistance should immediately begin to provide rapid processing of bird and mosquito specimens submitted for virus testing, and that would be made possible by the Mosquito Abatement for Safety and Health Act (S.2935) as introduced by Senators Breaux and Landrieu. The legislation could allow state and local governments to react more rapidly by providing funding to existing programs and states. Too much time has been lost in reporting results that could further direct control efforts. The point of surveillance is to detect the virus before it spreads to the human population; when weeks are required to report results the advantage of an early warning system is lost. Consequently, immediate preparation and funding are needed to allow state laboratories to continue testing dead birds submitted by citizens even after the virus activity has been detected in a particular parish. The additional data is vital in determining the exact location of the virus, which, in turn, allows a more direct assignment of abatement resources.

The Congress should also continue emergency funding for expanded surveillance, for testing and for state laboratories, which will play a role in early detection of the virus. My parish needs assurances that emergency supplemental funds will be available for additional mosquito control efforts should West Nile or any other mosquito-borne disease require a response beyond our local capabilities. This becomes particularly important when the disease is coupled with storms or man-made catastrophes that stretch available resources beyond their limits.

Mr. Chairman and Members of the Committee, this concludes my testimony. It was indeed a pleasure to be able to convey my thoughts on an important issue and a growing national health problem that will require a unified effort to combat. I want to thank each of you for your participation and am available to answer any questions you might have. Thank you.

PREPARED STATEMENT OF FAY W. BOOZMAN, M.D.

West Nile Virus infection is spreading rapidly; and, in Arkansas, it has reached epidemic levels in horses and birds. This is not unlike the experience in other states in the nation. In 1999, one state had evidence of the virus, while 12 states reported it in 2000, with 27 states in 2001 and now we are up to 42 states in 2002. Last year 48 human cases were reported in the U.S.; and, this year as of September 19, 1745 cases have been reported with 84 deaths.

Our neighboring state, Louisiana, had only one human case in 2001. This year, they have more than 260 human cases. Additionally, with 473 cases in Illinois as of September 20, we are concerned that migrating birds flying south will increase the disease burden on their way through Arkansas. It is likely that many of those birds will over winter in Southern Louisiana where the mosquito population may not die off due to cold weather.

This leads me to believe there is a real possibility that Arkansas will have a dramatic increase in human cases in 2003. We currently have 9 confirmed cases, with 18 more pending CDC confirmation.

We want to be ready to have an adequate surveillance and control program in place. Larviciding to reduce the mosquito population early in 2003 is a primary control activity that we want to emphasize in Arkansas. This mosquito abatement would be carried out at the county level. We are heartened by the financial assistance contained in the two bills before Congress, which will allow counties to implement these vital mosquito control programs.

At the state level, our primary needs are to expand laboratory capacity, and to augment and continue disease surveillance programs through testing. The coordination and evaluation called for in the two Congressional bills is necessary to ensure effective use of the mosquito abatement funding; however, we are concerned that more resources will be required than the proposed $10,000 in funding provided for the state.

CURRENT STATUS OF WEST NILE VIRUS ACTIVITY IN ARKANSAS

Human Cases

In Arkansas we currently have 9 CDC confirmed positive cases of West Nile Virus infection out of 408 blood and cerebrospinal fluid samples received as of September 19.

Included in the 408 patient samples are 18 suspect cases that have tested positive by IGM antibody capture ELISA testing at the ADH lab, but are awaiting a confirmation neutralization test at CDC.

There are currently 54 samples awaiting testing in the ADH laboratory.

The remainder of the samples from physicians tested negative, representing 328 patients.

The confirmed and suspect WNV human cases are from Pulaski, Union, Jefferson, Bradley, Arkansas, Desha, Crittenden, Monroe and Ouachita counties.

The Communicable Disease Nurse Specialists of the Arkansas Department of Health coordinate with physicians and hospitals testing for West Nile Virus and evaluate blood serum and cerebrospinal fluid samples. They determine demographic information on each patient, which includes age, sex, symptoms, onset date, the date blood was drawn, patient address, and any travel outside of the state where they may have been exposed.

Repeat samples are requested if the sample was drawn before antibodies were formed. It is necessary to evaluate the patients' symptoms and blood or CSF results before making a diagnosis.

Bird Testing

During 2002, as of September 20, the Livestock and Poultry Commission laboratory has reported 336 positive birds. Decomposed birds were not tested and 1245 birds were rejected because they were not suitable for analysis. Positive birds have been found in 48 of the 75 counties in Arkansas. Crows represented 22 percent of the positives, and 78 percent were blue jays. One owl, one hawk, one dove and one unidentified bird also tested positive for WNV infection.

Mosquito Testing

During 2002, mosquitoes were trapped at 34 different sites. Positive mosquitoes were found at five different locations around the state.

During 2002, as of September 19, there were five positive mosquito pools found in the counties of Pulaski, Jefferson and Desha. These positives were of the Culex species and were trapped with both Gravid and Light traps.

Surveillance in Horses

During 2002, as of September 20, there have been at least 130 horses tested for WNV and 56 have tested positive in 23 counties. The fatality rate is 39 percent, with 22 horses having died. The Arkansas Livestock and Poultry Commission conducts equine testing under a contract with the Department of Health.

During 2002, as of September 19, surveillance of horses for Eastern Equine Encephalitis has shown 20 cases in seven counties, with 19 of the 20 cases being fatal, a 95% fatality rate. This is the highest number of cases of EEE ever recorded in Arkansas and the onset was earlier in the year than has previously been seen. EEE is more of a threat to humans than WNV since the death rate in infected humans ranges from 30 - 70%.

Emergency Funding by the Governor

The Governor has released $1 million from his emergency funds to the 75 county judges for mosquito abatement. Health Department personnel developed a formula to equitably determine the amount of money each county would receive based on evidence of WNV in the county, its population and square miles.

The funding was distributed through the Arkansas Department of Emergency Management; however, the ADH facilitated a multi-agency review process of the applications for assistance. The University of Arkansas Cooperative Extension Service, and the Arkansas Plant Board were also involved in the application process.

The Governor also declared Arkansas a disaster area because of the WNV epidemic. This would make the state eligible for funding from the Federal Emergency Management Agency (FEMA) for mosquito control. The Arkansas Congressional delegation has written a letter of support for a Federal declaration from Health and Human Services Secretary Tommy Thompson.

County judges, city managers, city mayors and public works officials are involved in larvacidal treatment of mosquito breeding areas. They also direct adulticiding if human cases of WNV occur in their county. Local level Department Environmental Health Specialists also assisted in setting priorities for mosquito abatement by identifying mosquito breeding sites. Cooperative Extension Service Entomologists and county agents also assisted by advising county officials on mosquito control.

The majority of the 75 counties in Arkansas have little or no mosquito abatement capabilities. They need money for equipment, personnel training and chemicals. The estimated cost is $5 million for the state. The bills pending before Congress now could help address this need.

Centers for Disease Control Support

CDC assisted Arkansas by sending a team of Epidemiological Intelligence Service Professionals to Arkansas to assist in our disease surveillance program. They provided technical support in the area of electronically recording and tabulating data. We now have a database for human, bird and equine cases. We are also working on a GIS to pinpoint the location of positive cases.

CDC EIS officers also assisted the Department in identifying appropriate CDC contacts as questions and issues arose.

Laboratory samples are sent to CDC for confirmation. At CDC these samples are also tested for EEE, St. Louis Encephalitis and La Cross Encephalitis.

CDC has supported Arkansas by awarding a Cooperative Agreement to the state for $300,000 to cover the period from April 1, 2002 to April 1, 2003. Because of the dramatic spread of the disease during August of 2002 we were awarded supplemental funds of $398,000 for surveillance and to assist in controlling the disease.

CDC also provided television and radio public service announcements that could be customized for Arkansas.

Educational Activities

The medical community was sent special letters and faxes reminding them of the necessity to submit blood samples on all patients showing encephalitis or meningitis, proper preparation of the samples, and required patient information.

The Environmental Health Specialists were trained in mosquito abatement by the entomologist at the University of Arkansas Cooperative Extension Service. They were also trained in surveillance, mosquito speciation and mosquito trapping by the WNV Project Officer and by CDC personnel through special mosquito schools.

Outreach Activities

Local elected officials have been informed as human cases have been detected in their area. This contact with elected officials has been primarily by personnel at the local level.

ADH speakers frequently presented at clubs, civic organizations and other interested groups. The CDC power point presentation augmented with Arkansas data is routinely presented and is informative and gives a complete description of the disease and control measures.

We have printed and distributed 23,000 posters and brochures to the general public. We also printed coloring books for county fairs and schools.

Media relations have been excellent. The Health Director took the lead in appearing on television and radio. The State Epidemiologist appeared on talk shows and was interviewed by the television stations.

ADH has conducted three press conferences to release information on West Nile Virus.

Since August 5, 2002 the Arkansas Department of Health has issued over 20 press releases. Press releases and educational materials have been posted on our website and are available for the media and community to access the latest and most comprehensive information regarding West Nile in Arkansas. Updates are made as necessary. Media alerts are sent to statewide media outlets to inform them that the website has been updated.

The Public Information Office has emphasized the prevention message and precautions to avoid mosquito bites and to eliminate stagnant water in their area where mosquitoes can breed.

West Nile Virus Hotline

In order to answer our citizens' questions related to this disease, a telephone response center was established. The call center operated on a 24/7 basis with calls being answered by dedicated colleagues and the Department's Emergency Communication Center.

Because of the large number of phone calls from physicians, para-medical personnel and the general public it was necessary to have a Epidemiologist and M.D. on call 24/7. The on-call roster developed for a Bioterrorism response was effectively used and ensured that a professional was available.

Through September 11, 2002 the West Nile Hotline has answered 3,417 calls from the general public and health care providers.

Internal Communication Update

Internal Communication was emphasized to ensure that effective and timely information was provided from the WNV Project Team, to Business Unit Leaders, and others at the local level, including Hometown Health Leaders, Health Unit Administrators, Regional Leaders, Group Leaders, and Team Leaders.

Internal and external communication leaders worked as a team to ensure timely submission of press releases and communication between all entities before reports were made public.

Additional Needs

Funding is necessary to upgrade and improve our public health laboratory. The Department's laboratory needs to be upgraded to a Bio Safety Level 3 so live viruses can be analyzed. Also, our laboratory needs the capability to test for all types of arboviral encephalitis.

Abatement funding for the counties is estimated to require an additional $5 million.

The Livestock and Poultry Commission Laboratory test the birds, mosquitoes and horses on behalf of the Department of Health. Bird submission by the public exceeded expectations with more birds being received than the L&PC laboratory has capability to test. To expedite testing, a real time PCR testing device is needed.

PREPARED STATEMENT OF JOHN BARR

V.I. Technologies, Inc. (Vitex) is pleased today to have the opportunity to make the Committee aware of a fundamentally new and important approach to improving the safety of transfusion blood products.

Vitex applauds the rapid and intense investigation on the part of the CDC and FDA in dealing with the West Nile epidemic. We also applaud the creative approaches employed by the FDA with blood collectors and with companies such as Vitex to search for solutions to prevent the transmission of West Nile Virus by blood transfusion.

Unfortunately, West Nile Virus also highlights the vulnerability of the blood supply to an emerging pathogen. Current technology has limitations. Screening tests can literally take years to develop after a new pathogen has already entered the blood supply. The test must have the appropriate sensitivity. The new test is then implemented in all the community blood centers. Each new screening test can only test for a single pathogen. Other methods such as donor questionnaires can inadvertently prevent otherwise healthy donors from donating a unit of blood and constrain supply of blood components.

For too long our public health system has suffered through the cycle of bloodborne diseases causing illness and death followed by months of research to develop a screen that in turn diminishes potential blood donors. This soon need not be the case. At Vitex, we are developing a technology, now in phase 3 testing at the FDA, that will remove or inactivate disease-causing pathogens in red blood cells and break the cycle of responding to blood-borne diseases one at a time after they have caused harm or death.

VITEX

Vitex is a biotechnology company based in Massachusetts that is pioneering a new technology designed to improve the safety of red blood cell transfusions. The $INACTINE_{84}$ system for red blood cells produces a pathogen reduced red blood cell prepared using a combination of chemical inactivation and red cell purification. The system is currently in phase 3 testing, the final step in the clinical development program prior to filing for license approval with the FDA.

The $INACTINE_{84}$ system for red blood cells is a straightforward three step process. $INACTINE_{84}$ is added to a unit of red blood cells collected and manufactured just as it is today. The chemical remains in the unit overnight for the inactivation to occur. The $INACTINE_{84}$ is then removed using a process known as cell washing. The resulting unit of $INACTINE_{84}$-treated red blood cells is then ready for immediate transfusion or can be stored under standard blood bank conditions.

Pathogen Reduction: Vitex scientists in conjunction with outside collaborators have demonstrated inactivation of a broad spectrum of pathogens in full units of red blood cells using the $INACTINE_{84}$ system. These include both enveloped and non-enveloped viruses.

The $INACTINE_{84}$ system inactivates gram negative and gram positive bacteria. Further studies have demonstrated inactivation of parasites in units of red blood cells that can cause transmission of diseases such as malaria and Chagas' disease. The system has also has demonstrated robust removal of prions; an infectious form of the prion protein is thought to cause the human form of mad cow disease, variant Creutzfeldt—Jakob disease.

The $INACTINE_{84}$ system has demonstrated inactivation of lymphocytes. Based on these studies the system may have the potential to prevent graft versus host disease and other important immune complications such as alloimmunization. The system also removes other proteins that can cause transfusion reactions such as immunoglobulins, cytokines and other plasma proteins.

West Nile Virus Inactivation: Vitex has completed some experiments earlier this year with Dr. Fred Brown at the U.S.D.A. facility at Plum Island. Those studies demonstrated rapid inactivation of West Nile Virus in a full unit of red blood cells. These data were reported in August by Dr. Bernadette Alford, Executive Vice President of Vitex at the FDA workshop on the Safety and Efficacy of Methods for Reducing Pathogens in Cellular Blood Products.

West Nile Virus and Blood: As of Wednesday, September 18 the CDC reported 1,641 cases in the U.S. with over 80 deaths from an infection of West Nile Virus. An extensive investigation has been undertaken by the CDC and FDA to determine whether West Nile can be transmitted via organ donation and blood transfusion.

The CDC, in a telebriefing on Thursday, September 19 reported results of their ongoing investigation. An investigation in Georgia demonstrates that West Nile Virus transmission can occur via organ transplantation. A second investigation in Mississippi indicated that virus can survive in blood components and the CDC concluded that West Nile Virus ". . . probably can be transmitted by transfusion." (9/19/02, Update on West Nile Investigation)

Dr. Jesse Goodman, deputy director, FDA's Center for Biologics Evaluation and Research also participated in the briefing. Dr. Goodman concurred with the CDC's assessment that blood-borne transmission likely has occurred in some of these cases.

Dr. Goodman further outlined the actions the FDA is taking to reduce the potential risk of future blood-borne transmissions of West Nile Virus. These include product withdrawals of blood products that may carry a risk of transmission of West Nile Virus. In addition the FDA is providing guidance to blood collectors on new information to solicit from donors both before and after the donation. The FDA is also working with both blood collectors and the diagnostic testing industry to expedite the development of a blood screening test for West Nile Virus.

The FDA is exploring new approaches to improving blood safety. According to Dr. Goodman:

"Finally, there is another technology, called pathogen inactivation, which involves treatment of blood and blood products to kill potential infecting agents. This is a promising tool which FDA recently held a workshop on, that could potentially be used in our armamentarium as we address West Nile Virus threat. FDA is and has been working with manufacturers to evaluate the potential effectiveness and safety of this strategy, and will continue to discuss this specifically with respect to West Nile Virus." (9/19/02 Update on West Nile Investigation)

Vitex shares Dr. Goodman's view of the potential of pathogen inactivation technologies such as the $INACTINE_{84}$ system to improve the safety of red blood cells. A broad spectrum inactivation system such as INACTINE(TM) has the potential to improve the safety of red blood cell transfusions. We further believe the

INACTINE$_{8\&}$ system may prevent the transmission of West Nile Virus in a unit of red blood cells. A broad spectrum pathogen inactivation system also offers the promise of inactivation of future emerging challenges to the safety of the blood supply.

Implementation of Pathogen Inactivation Technology in the Health Care System: Over the past several years, Congress has recognized the inadequacy of the formulas for reimbursing health care providers for the cost of blood and blood products and for the use of new technologies. The rapid spread of West Nile Virus shows how essential it is to introduce new preventive technologies, such as pathogen inactivation for red blood cells, with a sense of urgency that matches the speed with which these new emerging threats attack the public's health. We urge Congress to ensure that adequate reimbursement is made a priority for new blood safety technologies such as the INACTINE$_{8\&}$ system so that the patients can immediately benefit by their widespread adoption.

VITEX appreciates this opportunity to inform the Congress about the promise pathogen inactivation presents to improve the safety of the blood supply and to protect public health.

LETTER FROM SARA C. YERKES, INTERNATIONAL CODE COUNCIL (ICC)

September 26, 2002

THE HONORABLE EDWARD M. KENNEDY
Chairman
Committee on Health, Education, Labor and Pensions
SD–644 Dirksen Senate Office Building
Washington, D.C. 20510–6300

DEAR SENATOR KENNEDY:

The International Code Council (ICC) commends you and all the Members of the Senate Committee on Health, Education, Labor and Pensions and the Subcommittee on Oversight of Government Management, Restructuring and the District of Columbia on holding a joint hearing on the West Nile Virus health threat.

ICC is a not-for-profit organization whose mission is to promulgate a comprehensive and compatible regulatory system for the built environment through consistent performance-base regulations that are effective, efficient and meet government, industry and public needs. ICC develops the International Codes, a single comprehensive and coordinated functional set of codes governing building construction.

ICC respectfully requests that this statement be included in the record of the Joint Committee Hearing held on September 24, 2002 by the two committees mentioned above.

The International Codes can play a key role in the fight against the West Nile Virus. ICC has over 190 years of collective experience in developing comprehensive and coordinated codes for building construction. To date there are 44 states enforcing one or more of the International Codes. Approximately 97 percent of cities, counties and states are using documents published by ICC and its members. For more information on ICC or the International Codes, please visit our website: **www.intlcode.org.**

On September 24, 2002 the Committees heard testimony from the medical and health research communities. The spread of the West Nile Virus has become a primary concern to health officials across the country. ICC and its 50,000 individual members, 9,000 cities, 50 states and over 80 trade and professional organizations can help combat this problem.

Building codes that have been adopted by local governments can play a key role in the fight against the West Nile Virus and other mosquito-borne diseases. The best way to prevent the spread of the West Nile Virus is to attack the breeding ground of the mosquitoes that could potentially carry the disease. Areas of stagnant water should be eliminated. In addition, screens over windows and doors should be "big tight." Most people willingly maintain their properties according to health standards, but in some cases, certain guidelines must be enforced. The ICC's International Codes can help. The International Property Maintenance Code® (IPMC) can assist local officials in enforcing the cleanup of existing properties. The IPMC® can combat the spread of mosquitoes and mosquito-borne viruses.

Local jurisdictions can contribute to the mitigation of this virus by adopting and enforcing the International Property Maintenance Code® (IPMC). The provisions in Chapter 3 of this code, when enforced by local jurisdictions, can assist in the slowing down of the spread of this virus and other infectious diseases by requiring that property owners meet certain minimum standards in the upkeep of their property. Requirements such as: (1) the property must be graded and drained so that there will be no accumulation of stagnant water; (2) a requirement for the proper drainage of roofs and gutters; (3) a requirement that addresses the accumulation and disposal of garbage; and (4) requirements that address the extermination of insects. The provisions of this code apply to both residential and commercial structures.

Other provisions of the IPMC® are also useful to local jurisdictions. The code also addresses vacant structures and land, requiring that these properties not "cause a blighting problem or adversely affect the public health and safety,." It addresses weeds and excessive plant growth. All of these sections of the IPMC® provide local jurisdictions the enforcement tools they need in order to require property owners to clean up unsanitary conditions on their property that harbor the growth and proliferation of the mosquito population.

Local jurisdictions have a powerful and useful tool in the IPMC® to assist in the fight against the West Nile Virus. Working in conjunction with local health departments, they can help ensure the health and safety of their communities. Currently the IPMC® is being enforced in twenty-five states. Three states, Michigan, New York and Oklahoma, have adopted the code statewide. In the other states, the code was adopted by local jurisdictions.

In conclusion, ICC offers its assistance to Congress in finding the best means to protect the public against the threat of the West Nile Virus. We urge the Members to consider including ICC in the programs to be operated through the Centers for Disease Control and Prevention program as called for in S. 2935, "Mosquito Abatement for Safety and Health Act."

Thank you for the opportunity to comment on this important national health problem. Please feel free to contact me if I may be of any assistance to your Committee.

Sincerely,

SARA C. YERKES
Vice President of Public Policy

○